MW01275736

IT IS IN YOUR HANDS:
EMOTIONAL FREEDOM TECHNIQUE

The Power to Eliminate Stress, Anxiety, and All Negative Emotions

Sobeida Salomon, Ph.D.

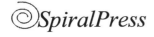*SpiralPress*

Ambler, Pennsylvania

Disclaimer. The information contained in this book is for educational purposes and it is not intended to be a substitute for medical or psychological professional health care. If professional medical or psychological advice or other expert assistance is required, the services of a competent professional should be sought. The author or the publisher does not assume any responsibility or any liability, explicitly or implied, on the results or the consequences of using the information contained in this book . The author or the publisher makes no warranty of any kind with regard to the material, and shall not be liable for errors contained therein, or direct, indirect, special, incidental, or consequential damages in connection with the furnishing, performance, or use of this material. **If you do not wish to be bound by the foregoing, please return this book to the publisher for a full refund.**

IT IS IN YOUR HANDS: EMOTIONAL FREEDOM TECHNIQUE
The Power to Eliminate Stress, Anxiety, and All Negative Emotions.

Published by *SpiralPress*, a division of *HydroScience Inc.*

SpiralPress
1217 Charter Lane
Ambler, PA 19002
Email: hydroscience@earthlink.net
http://home.earthlink.net/~hydroscience
SAN 299-3074

Library of Congress Cataloging-in-Publication Data

Salomon, Sobeida, 1953-
It is in your hands : emotional freedom technique : the power to eliminate stress, anxiety, and all negative emotions / Sobeida Salomon.
p. cm.
Includes bibliographical references and index.
ISBN 978-0-9655643-6-6 (pbk. : alk. paper)
1. Emotions. 2. Acupuncture points. 3. Stress (Psychology) 4. Mind and body therapies.
I. Title.

RC489.E45S25 2007
616.89'16--dc22
2007026529

Printed in the United States of America
ISBN: 978-0-9655643-6-6

I dedicate this book to Sergio, for his constant encouragement through every step of my life.

*"Mistakes and shortcomings of the past shall have no more dominion over you; **in your hands** is the key which opens up the way to all **freedom** and accomplishment."*

Henry Thomas Hamblin
(Dynamic Thought. The Yogi Pub. Soc., Chicago, 1923).

CONTENTS

1.

IT IS IN YOUR HANDS

Eliminate All of Your Negative Emotions

You have in your hands a book that will change your life. It Is in Your Hands: Emotional Freedom Technique (EFT) is an introduction to a revolutionary psychological therapeutic method. Also in your hands is the power to eliminate all negative emotions, including: stress, anxiety, fears, phobias, past traumas, substance abuse and all addictions. You no longer have to go through months of expensive and usually ineffective, conventional "talk therapies." In a matter of minutes, you can be free from any negative emotional or psychological difficulty that in the past has haunted you or prevented you from reaching your full potential. EFT puts in your hands the power to eliminate all negative emotions and live a joyful, blissful life. It is simple, effective, and most importantly, it is free!

You are probably searching for new alternatives to improve your life; for simple ways to clear those emotional patterns that have been with you for as long as you can remember, or for methods that will allow you to use your own natural healing energies. In the privacy of your own home or office, you can relieve any stress or discomfort that is preventing you from preparing a business presentation or public speaking engagement. You can quickly eliminate any fears or phobias you have been carrying since childhood. You can relieve any feelings of discomfort or anger towards a coworker or a relative and do more productive work. You can dissolve any past resentment with respect to your close family members or relatives and in fact enjoy an unusually stress-free holiday reunion.

You can eliminate your undesirable bad habits or addictions that prevent you from having a peaceful and enjoyable life. With EFT you can re-create your life the way it is supposed to be: healthy, happy, abundant, peaceful, and prosperous.

Psychological and self-help literature constantly emphasizes the need for us to work on our negative patterns, to have a positive attitude in life, to overcome our emotional problems, and to move forward. We all see the benefit on this new way of thinking and behaving, but we are confronted with the problem of not knowing how to change, how to move to the next step. EFT offers that alternative. This new technique is the therapy of the new century. You do not have to believe that it will work; it simply does! Whether you believe in it or not, EFT is simple, effective, and easy to apply. It is a powerful technique to eliminate stress, fear, anger, frustrations, anxiety, phobias, trauma, addiction or any other form of negative emotion. You can apply it to yourself and obtain results very fast. The only thing it requires is a few minutes of your time, your hands, and the desire to free yourself from unwanted negative emotions. These attributes made Emotional Freedom Technique an outstanding self-help protocol that professionals can use with their clients, and people can easily apply towards their own personal growth.

Emotional Freedom Technique (EFT) and Thought Field Therapies (TFT) access the body's energy meridian system to release the negative energy attached to a particular negative emotion. The energy meridian system is a natural network of energy pathways circulating through the body. EFT uses the same principles of energy therapies, such as the ancient healing art of acupuncture, except that EFT does not require needles and it heals psychological problems.

You use your own hands to stimulate the major meridian points in a specific sequence by tapping at each point with your fingers. While you tap at each meridian point, you need to focus your mind on the specific problem or emotion that you want to eliminate. The purpose of the tapping series is to reestablish the normal flow of energy in your body.

EFT was designed and developed by Gary Craig who based his new approach on Dr. Roger Callahan's development of Thought Feel Therapy (TFT). TFT is the outcome of a recent extraordinary scientific discovery that found that the cause of negative emotions is not the memory of a traumatic event, but the negative energy entangled around the memory. This discovery showed that by releasing this energy, the negative emotion is instantly eliminated. Thousands of people have reported being relieved from past traumas and negative feelings that previously required months, or even years, of sometimes-unsuccessful conventional treatment.

The fundamental theory of TFT states that "The cause of all negative emotions is a disruption in the body's energy system." It is a simple but fundamental principle that radically departs from the traditional way in which psychology treats emotional problems.

The premise of EFT is that when we experience fear, stress, or any other unwanted emotion, the flow of energy in our body is interrupted. This blockage causes an imbalance in our energy system thus producing an emotional response. By stimulating the various body end meridian points, the normal energy flow is reestablished and the emotional response that was experienced before is eradicated: the fear, the anxiety, or the stress we were experiencing disappears and all that is left is the memory of the event. All you need is to lo learn the location of a selected set of meridian end points, the use of your hands to stimulate these points for a few minutes, and the ability to concentrate and feel a particular negative emotion you want to eliminate. It is that simple!

EFT is in the process of constant development. As with any new field of knowledge, EFT/TFT has been received with skepticism by main-stream psychology, which stands to lose the most to a new therapeutic technique that, unlike most conventional ones, offers a permanent cure to the patient. However, new rigorous scientific research is slowly being published in main-stream science journals confirming the positive effects of EFT/TFT. People around the world are using EFT and reporting, not only complete resolution to their emotional problems, but also remarkable improvement on various physical afflictions.

This book is divided into eight chapters. Before you apply EFT, I recommend you read the book in order, familiarize yourself with the different tapping points, learn the exact location of each point, the order of tapping, and the construction of the affirmations. Detailed pictures are provided to help you memorize the points. Then apply EFT to a particular negative emotion you wish to eliminate. Many negative emotions are eliminated within minutes; what remains is just the memory of the past event, but no emotion attached to it. Other deeply ingrained chronic patterns require several sessions. You must persist on its application until all aspects of the problem have been eradicated. Many suggestions are given about how to treat specific addictions or problems. Ideas are provided about the extensive use of EFT to systematically eliminate all of your negative emotions and their ramifications. The result is a new person, free from all past negative patterns, and free to live life the way he or she wants. However, this time you are in control of your life, not your past traumas and restrictions. Be persistent and you will be gratified with the results.

We emphasize that EFT is not a substitute for professional psychological treatment. Many deep psychological and violent traumas require professional help. Also, for many severe mental disorders it is recommended to use professional help to get you started in your own use of EFT. This is specially true if you are not used to self analysis, or you are not aware of your common patterns. Many psychologists and counselors are beginning to use EFT in their professional practice. Professional care with the aid of EFT will give an added advantage. Whatever treatment you are currently using, EFT will not interfere with it, but enhance it and may in fact help you achieve its goals.

"When you are grieving, when you compulsively overeat, or when you are anxious, there is a perturbation in a Thought Field. The perturbation holds the information that governs these and all negative or disturbing emotions."

Roger Callahan.

2.

Thought Field Therapy and Emotional Freedom Technique

A Cure for Emotional Problems

Thought Field Therapy (TFT) and Emotional Freedom Techniques (EFT) are radically different psychotherapy techniques to treat emotional problems. These techniques go beyond the conventional top down treatments. The traditional approach is well known by all of us who at one point or another in our life have sought out psychological counseling. The client and therapist come together with a mutual understanding; the client will discuss his emotional concerns and the therapist, guided by her psychological theoretical perspectives, will present alternatives to the client to deal with his problems. The treatment lasts months, if not years, of therapist-client interaction. It usually brings psychological pain and demands endurance on the part of the client, as he has to revive the series of traumatic events that led him to seek psychological help. The treatment may cost thousands of dollars. For the therapist, it implies dealing with frustration and despair to see the client making very slow progress if at all.

EFT/TFT techniques eliminate the need of this relationship by offering the client an instrument to solve his emotional problems on his own. The power and control are now literally in the hands of the client. These therapeutic techniques are very effective, simple to apply, and inexpensive. Their results can be observed and evaluated immediately. As with most new developments, it requires an open mind, because it is a radical departure from the conventional methods of treating emotional problems.

This book offers a self-guided procedure that empowers the client. It provides the tools to heal difficult emotional problems, such as emotional traumas, anxiety, addictions, phobias, anger, guilt, fears, insecurities, negativity, and physical pain associated with these. EFT/TFT is based on the use of the body's energy system. They are very easy to learn and apply. The procedure consists in tapping with your fingers on specific points on your body, while thinking about the negative emotion you want to eliminate.

It is important to clarify that this therapeutic technique will not delete the memory of the event that caused the trauma, but it will eliminate the emotional reaction that surrounds the event. In other words, the treatment will set you free from the emotional pain associated with the memory. You will feel free to be yourself and to act and respond to situations in a calm and objective maner. You will take control of your feelings, instead of being dominated by them.

Clearing your negative emotions is an important part of health and happiness. When we do not work in our behavioral patterns, our emotions tend to reemerge every time we face similar situations that re-stimulate us. To establish an analogy it is as if we play a scratched CD that repeats itself over and over again, without our control. We find ourselves not knowing why certain distressful situations keep repeating themselves. Thus, we automatically react in the same manner, without control over our emotions. EFT/TFT break this behavioral pattern. In some cases the treatment is so effective that the client has difficulty accepting she has been permanently cured. She believes the familiar pattern will return at any time when in fact she has been cured.

The fundamental element to be successful with EFT/TFT is to be in touch with the negative feelings that are causing the physical or emotional reaction in our body. By focusing on the negative feeling while tapping, the energies trapped around the traumatic event will be freed. Whether it is   fear, anger, resentment, phobia, trauma, anxiety, guilt, grief, or physical pain, TFT/EFT brings emotional stability and well being by reestablishing emotional balance.

A Personal Experience with TFT/EFT

EFT/TFT techniques came to my life at a crucial time. I was working as a therapist for an institution that served court adjudicated youth. It was a half way house for girls, ages twelve to seventeen. This was also their last hope before entering the justice system. The girls came from different parts of a city with a myriad of social and emotional problems. Many of the girls were victims of physical, emotional, and sexual abuse. As expected, they harbored anger, resentment, mistrust, sadness, and in many cases uncontrollable rage. This institution offered a comprehensive approach to the girls' well being. It was a safe haven away from the turbulence of their home and community environment. At that time, this center was undergoing serious financial, administrative, and program restructuring problems.

There were many seemingly unresolvable issues of personnel management and relationships. The staff's morale was at an all-time low. The place was in total chaos.

Almost overnight, I was appointed director of the center. As a consequence, this chaos became my responsibility. The working environment was toxic and I was in the line of fire. I felt extremely tense, trying to work with my own feelings of desperation, as well as having to present an optimistic approach to encourage the teachers, the general staff, the students, and their families. At the same time, I learned that the center was going to be eliminated, closing its doors for good. The students had to be relocated and all of the staff members, including me, were going to be laid off. Faced with all of these misfortunes, and overwhelmed by stress, one of the psychologists of the center suggested to me that I try an unorthodox technique that could help me alleviate the pressure I was feeling. It was an extraordinary gift he gave me. In a very short time, EFT helped me regain my confidence. I also helped several of the staff members to deal with the series of traumatic events we all went through. I stood behind the center supporting the staff and the girls with courage and equanimity until it closed its doors. EFT helped me immensely to cope with many distressful feelings remaining after my departure from the center. I found myself without a job, on Christmas, holding strong feelings of betrayal, anger, and discontent toward the institution. I felt appalled knowing that the center had jeopardized not only the employees' stability but also the safety and care of the students. It was a real test for EFT effectiveness. Several years have passed since then, I eliminated all those negative feelings, and I have continued to use EFT/TFT with my clients and myself with a resounding success in most cases.

3.

The Origins of Thought Field Therapy (TFT) and Emotional Freedom Technique (EFT)

New Discovery with Ancient Roots

This is a new and constantly changing therapeutic field attracting not only specialists in different areas but also regular people, like you, who are interested in alternative curative methods. Thought Field Therapy (TFT) was introduced by Dr. Roger Callahan, who in turn credits the development of this new therapeutical approach to ancient Chinese medicine, acupuncture and acupressure. These methods are well known in the western world today. They are ancient techniques that work with what the Chinese call the channels or energy meridians, which are present in our body system.

Whereas acupuncture uses needles inserted into different points of the body or meridian points, acupressure uses firm pressure with the fingers to stimulate key points on the surface of the skin activating the body's autonomic curative capacity (Forem, J. and Shimer, S., 1999). They both work with the body's life force energy to effectively clear energy blockages reestablishing the normal flow of energy. In developing TFT, Callahan (2001) used the principles of Chinese medicine as well as new developments in the applied kinesiology field pioneered by G. Goodheart (1964).

It could be said that TFT was born in 1980 during an accidental discovery that completely revolutionized the treatment of psychological disturbances. Callahan had exhausted all of the available techniques to solve a problem and was experimenting with an open mind with new techniques. He found by accident that by stimulating an energy meridian associated with a particular psychological disturbance, the energy attached to the disturbance was released and an instant cure was obtained (Callahan, 2001). Dr. Callahan is a former professor of psychology, who had grown frustrated with the ineffectiveness of most psychotherapy treatments. He was treating a patient named Mary for over a year, who had a severe water phobia. He tried all conventional psychotherapeutic techniques he knew: Rational-emotive therapy, client-centered therapy, cognitive therapy, behavior therapy, hypnosis, relaxation training, biofeedback, systematic desensitization. Everything failed. During one session one day, Mary told him of the intense stomach pain she felt when in proximity of a swimming pool. Dr. Callahan had been reading much about the energy meridians as described in ancient acupuncture studies, and remembered that under the eye is located the end point of a meridian that connects with the stomach. It occurred to him to ask Mary to tap with her fingers under the eye. After two minutes the patient was cured. This was a permanent cure. In other words, Mary's fears were instantly and forever gone. This was a patient for whom even the thought of water made her sick. Within minutes of treatment she was by the swimming pool splashing water on her face.

He continued with his research, replicating and refining the "Taping technique while tuning the mind on the afflicting emotion." He realized that he had developed a new, totally unconventional, fast, and effective approach to cure emotional problems. Through his practice he concluded that different emotional problems needed different "taping points" to stimulate the body energy or meridian associated with the emotion. He developed what he called specific "algorithms" that involved tuning the mind into a negative emotion and simultaneously taping different parts of the body in a distinctive sequence. Each algorithm was prescribed for a specific emotional problem.

To evaluate the success of his technique he uses a ten-point scale before doing any treatment. For instance, he asked his patients to evaluate the magnitude of his/her phobia. While the patient was thinking about it, the patient evaluated his emotional condition on a subjective scale from one to ten, with ten being the maximum discomfort and one being totally calmed and relaxed. In this way the practitioner, or the user if one is applying a self treatment, can determine the effectiveness of the technique. For instance, if the client reports a number eight prior to treatment, and after the treatment it decreases to five, this is an indication that the treatment is being effective. However, the treatment must be reapplied until the user reports no negative emotion, or a number one on the scale.

As with any new discovery, Callahan's contribution has been criticized by main stream psychology. This is a procedure that would make many traditional talk therapies redundant. Critics contend that after two decades TFT has not been substantiated by controlled statistical and scientific experimentation and the results published in peer-reviewed psychology journals. Research on controlled experiments is beginning to appear in scientific literature, especially in regards to derivative methods of TFT, such as emotional freedom techniques (EFT) described later.

TFT as well as many other alternative medicine procedures have been slow in attracting the attention of main stream science. The reason why TFT has not been validated is the same as why many natural herbal supplements have not been validated by the pharmaceutical industry. For instance, the powerful and very profitable pharmaceutical industry is not interested in financing research that would validate the healing effects of St. John's Wort for the treatment of depression. The natural herb costs about 4 dollars per bottle and appears to produce the same results as those of prescription antidepressants that cost over 100 dollars (Lecrubier, et al. 2002; Sahelian, 2007). Furthermore, the natural herb has no side effects, while the prescription drugs may have health threatening consequences. Why finance research that would make expensive chemicals obsoletes?

Until more quantitative reports on the effectiveness of TFT techniques are available, the public must rely on qualitative reports, which are equally valid. Callahan's books and the Internet sites for TFT and EFT are filled with anecdotal reports on the positive effects of these methods. People from all over the world report good results. This should be a motivation to try them. As I have stated before, measure the risks and costs involved, which in this case are negligible, and try them yourself. Accept only what you have thoroughly demonstrated by your own experimentation.

The Basis of Thought Field Therapy

Callahan's discovery reaffirms the age long understanding that the human body is a complex electrochemical system of metabolic and psychic processes. The driving force of these processes is what the ancient healers from Hawaii, the Kahunas named Mana, which is given different names by other traditions (Serrano, 2007). For nearly five thousand years, the Chinese culture has advanced and refined an elaborate acupuncture medicine system. This system postulates that the human body is crossed by a network of energy pathways, called meridians, where the *chi* energy (life vital force) circulates. This energy and its associated meridians are invisible to the human eye, although they have been detected by modern scientific instrumentation (Swingle et al., 2004). Each meridian pathway crosses a particular set of internal organs and ends at specific points on the surface of the skin. Acupuncture treatments use needles inserted at a meridian end point associated with a specific diseased organ. Many theories attempt to explain the reason why these treatments are very effective. One states that a disease results from a blockage in the body's energy system and that by the action of a good electrical conductor (i.e., the needle) the energy blockage is released and a harmonious flow of energy is restored throughout the body.

Callahan defined a Thought Field as a fundamental intangible unit or structure containing large amounts of mental information. Callahan's Thought Field corresponds to the Kahunas thought seed, which contains feelings, pictures, and other sensations related to a particular memory (Serrano, 2007). This seed is attached to various amounts of Mana energy according to the intensity with which the memory was initially produced. If the memory relates to a stressful event, it may have been improperly rationalized and incorrectly stored in the subconscious and with unusually large amounts of Mana attached to it. Large amounts of energy stored in a particular thought seed or cluster of thought seeds disrupt the normal flow of energy in the energy meridian passing through the cluster. By stimulating the end point of the corresponding energy meridian the amount of energy abnormally stored in the Thought Field, or thought seed, is released thus restoring the normal flow of energy. The human fingers may act as the electrical conductor that discharges the trapped energy.

The effect might be similar to that of discharging a battery that powers a recorder. The recorder plays a message over and over. When the battery power is discharged, it can no longer drive the messages stored in the recorder. The messages are not deleted, but they are no longer played.

For this effect to be possible, the patient needs to tune into the distressing feeling or memory, which accesses the specific Thought Field, while tapping the associated set of meridian end points. This process restores the normal flow of energy, but does not delete the memory itself, which will remain in the Thought Field, but will not longer trigger a distressful response when recalled. According to ancient Eastern medicine, mental and physical health is characterized by a normal (not too low or not too high) flow of energy through the human network of meridians (Eden and Feinstein, 1998; Teeguarden, 1978). Callahan's main contribution has been to extend the age long knowledge of acupuncture and acupressure to the realm of psychological disturbances.

4.

Emotional Freedom Technique (EFT)

Improved Generalized Procedure

Callahan's Thought Field Therapy (TFT) constitutes the first and most extensive set of treatment techniques in this line of work. Each TFT treatment is designed for a specific psychological disturbance (Callahan, 2001). The user needs to diagnose the type of problem to treat and then consult the specific treatment therapy, or algorithm, to use. The treatment itself might be done in minutes and the rate of success is very high. Each treatment involves tuning into the distressful feeling or memory while repetitively tapping with your fingers on a set of meridian end points. The sequence of points to tap must be done in the specified order.

Subsequent to Callahan's development of TFT, a number of variants have been proposed in what have been called Meridian Energy Therapies (MET). One of the most successful improvements of the original TFT has been proposed by Gary Craig, who developed a single generalized treatment technique for all psychological disturbances. Craig called this improvement Emotional Freedom Techniques (EFT).

Attracted to the possibility of the five-minute-phobia cures taught by Callahan, Gary Craig took Callahan's training. Although he was very impressed with the results obtained by the new techniques, he was also critical of the rigidity of Callahan's different algorithms which have to be applied in an exact sequence of tapping the points in order to treat a specific emotion. Craig expressed concerns that in many instances it is very difficult and even impossible to separate our emotions. One specific situation can elicit, at the same time, feelings of anger and sadness, or the event may consist of many other emotions that could be very difficult to separate. Craig stated that in such cases Callahan's treatment would not be effective because it requires a precise taping protocol to address a very specific emotion.

With this in mind, Craig set himself the task to make Callahan's TFT treatment more comprehensive, easier to remember, and simpler to apply. He developed an alternative treatment procedure: instead of using precise energy meridian end points to address a specific emotion, the user now applies a comprehensive and inclusive approach that involves taping all the meridians points, independently of the emotion. In that way, by default you will always tap the energy points associated with the emotion and will obtain positive results. He called his new approach Emotional Freedom Technique (EFT).

The most important contribution of EFT is simplicity. There is only one treatment, regardless of the disturbance to treat. This treatment covers all of the end points and there is no need to memorize complex sequences. In the following pages I summarize the simplified EFT method. I remark that this is not a substitute for professional therapeutic help, which should be consulted in cases of severe complexes or very deep fixations. An initial set of visits to a good therapist, or better, a specialized TFT/EFT therapist, can help pinpoint the trouble areas to look into. For many problems involving our daily stresses, fears, insomnia, guilt and grief, one can use these techniques by itself with great success.

The core of his new technique rests on the belief that **"The cause of all negative emotions is a disruption in the body's energy system."** This implies that fears, phobias, anger, anxiety, depression, grief, guilt, worry, traumatic memories, the total scope of negative emotions has the same source: **an interference in the body's energy system**. This is a simple statement with profound implications; it is based on the fact that all of our emotional problems can be handled and solved when the normal flow of energy in our body is re-established.

The following analogy can assist in the understanding of this concept. Picture a system powered by energy, for instance any electrical appliance that works properly but for some reason or another a fuse had burned inside. As a result, the appliance does not work, its energy had been blocked producing a dysfunction in the system. This problem can only be solved when the broken connection is reestablished and the energy flows freely. Another analogy to aid in the understanding of this fundamental concept involves picturing a string of Christmas lights which are all connected in series by the same electrical cord. If one of the bulbs burns, the electricity cannot circulate and none of the bulbs will work until the malfunctioning bulb is replaced and the energy starts to circulate freely again. The equilibrium has been reestablished.

The same principle applies to us. When our energy becomes blocked by a negative emotion, it produces a disruption in our body's energy system. Our energy cannot flow freely and that causes an emotional response of fear, anger, stress, anxiety, panic, etc. When we release the energy blockage by tapping through the specific meridian ending points, we reestablish the energy flow and permanently liberate ourselves from the negative emotion that was affecting our system. In this way, we can stop being the victims of our emotions and be free to be the person we were meant to be all along: confident, creative, intelligent, sensitive, outspoken, assertive, and calm. These are just some of our qualities that are hindered when there is a blockage in our natural flow of energy.

Martha's Case

The following case illustrates how a dysfunctional family environment could limit our personal and professional development for the rest of our lives. In this process we negatively affect, not only ourselves, but also the lives of those we interact with.

A 25-year-old client that I will call Martha came to see me to seek counseling for a problem that she has had for as long as she could remember. She complained about not being able to write well, and every time she had to write a report for her classes or a simple note to a friend she felt very anxious and very insecure. Her problem was exacerbated if somebody was looking at her while she was writing, such as a colleague watching her computer screen from behind. Her feelings of inadequacy did not seem to bear any relationship with her formal education. Martha had a degree in science, she succeeded in graduate school, and now she was offered a new position in a pharmaceutical company that required constant report writing. She felt so insecure of her ability to write that she started having panic attacks. She was not able to sleep or to concentrate on any activity and was having second thoughts about accepting the new job.

I started her treatment by asking her when was the first time she became conscious of the problem. In the beginning, she was unable to identify that time, but after three sequences of EFT, pictures of her childhood came to her mind. She recalled the main events in her life when she internalized that she was not good at writing and she started to believe that she was never going to succeed professionally. Martha's parents were from Asia and she grew up with very strict rules. Education was extremely important to her family. Her parents believed that it was better to be home schooled than to go to the local public school to waste precious time. According to Martha's recollection, her parents used to say "The alphabet must be learned with blood," expressing the belief that a disciplined environment was the best for learning. They set the task to teach her to read and write. Each time she made a mistake, her mother would hit her on her head, sometimes so severely that her nose bled. Her mother also accompanied the physical abuse with denigrating verbal abuse. She constantly said to Martha that she was good for nothing, that she was never going to learn how to write or to succeed at anything in life. Interestingly, her sister was also taught at home and was subjected to the same abuses, but she did not develop the same problem and contrary to Martha, her sister grew up to be a confident research professor. This proves that similar environments do not necessarily produce the same results.

According to the main premises of EFT, when Martha was experiencing the anxiety of learning to write, her energy system was disrupted. That energy disruption was what caused her negative emotional reaction to writing. The physical and verbal abuses undoubtedly contributed to Martha's traumatic reaction to writing, but according to EFT, they are not the *cause*. This is a radical departure from traditional psychology, because according to EFT Martha's negative emotions (fear, anxiety, and panic) were not caused by the memory of her traumatic experience of her mother's abuses when teaching her to write. *Instead, the cause of her writing problems was her reaction to the traumatic events she experienced.* Specifically, the improper rationalization that identifies "writing," or more precisely "making a writing mistake," with the fear of physical and verbal punishment. This internalization was done with the aid of enormous emotional energy in the form of pain and shock of the punishment. This energy remains attached to the memory. Even though Martha is consciously aware that a writing mistake will no longer bring such punishment, her unconscious mind is unable to believe this. Each time the thought of writing emerges, the old program is triggered with the same energy and intensity with which it was recorded during childhood. By clearing the energy associated with the original event, the old program will no longer limit her. Many other traumas associated with the original experience will at the same time be cleared.

Traditional therapies would have treated Martha by inviting her to relive the original incident several times over a period of weeks, months, or years, thus causing enormous emotional pain. In this process the therapist would assist Martha in rationalizing the event, to let go of the pain, and to understand that it is no longer relevant. This objective is often partially achieved or not at all. In most circumstances the patient will learn to manage the distress, but most traditional psychological therapies will not render a cure. In contrast, the EFT treatment focused on releasing the energy blockage and negative energy attached to the memory. In EFT treatment, the only reference to the original memory is to investigate the cause, but the client does not have to relive the memory. For Martha this was done in two sessions of 45 minutes achieving a complete cure. Martha decided to accept her new job and she is doing well. She recently told me that each time she feels anything mildly associated with her writing, she uses EFT techniques on her own, thus relieving any fears. The EFT therapy did not remove Martha's memory. However, by removing the negative energy associated with it, the memory of the event no longer has any power over her. Conventional therapy addresses the memory of the abuse but for EFT they are not the cause, only contributors to the trauma.

The advantage of this technique of total emotional freedom resides on the capacity that each and every one of us has to apply it. This can easily be done without the need of painful, long, and expensive therapy. We can work in clearing up our negative emotions in the privacy of our own homes or at any time we determine appropriate. We can clear ourselves of past traumatic experiences that limit our lives. We can eliminate self-destructive messages that control the way we think and act, which prevent us from achieving our total potential.

There are many evidences that attest to the effectiveness of (EFT). This technique has helped thousands all around the world. Mental health professionals, general physicians, physical therapists, and alternative medicine practitioners are using EFT in their everyday practices. Thousands of cases attesting to its success have been submitted to Craig's Internet site. However, the most remarkable aspect of EFT protocol is the fact that regular people like you can use it too and obtain the same benefits.

In addition to the overwhelming qualitative evidence on

the effectiveness of EFT treatments, EFT techniques are beginning to be verified in controlled scientific experiments with promising results. A ground-breaking publication (Wells et al., 2003) demonstrated the effectiveness of EFT in treating animal phobias. Swingle et al. (2004) showed that there are measurable physiological effects resulting from the successful application of EFT treatments. The research subjects received a pretreatment and post treatment assessment of 19 brain locations (i.e., a "brain map") that used the QEEG (Quantitative Electroencephalograph) to convert brain waves to quantitative values that reflect the frequency and amplitude of brain wave activity at various brain locations. The results indicated that neurological psychology may be used to measure the effects of EFT treatments, but more importantly that the effects of a successful treatment corresponds to true physiological responses and not just self suggestion. Another important point, is that this study corroborated the physical responses parallel to EFT psychological treatments. Many users of EFT have reported success in the treatment of *physical* ailments.

EFT only requires that you follow a simple protocol of taping points, a synchronization with the negative emotion that you want to eradicate, and a few minutes of your time. To determine the degree of emotional relief you have obtained it is paramount that prior to the treatment you attune your thoughts to the negative emotion and ask yourself the following question: on the Subjective Units of Distress (SUD) scale from 1 to 10, with 1 being no discomfort or emotional pain at all and 10 being maximum pain and unbearable emotional discomfort, how strong do I feel about this emotion? The number you assign will be your reference indicator to judge your progress with the treatment. If after the first treatment this number has not come down to 1, you will need to re-apply the tapping treatment. EFT is so extremely effective that in many cases it only takes one round of taping to get our emotions from an 8 to a 1. In other cases, some extra rounds of the complete taping protocol will be necessary to totally clear the traumatic experience or negative emotion. If you consider the fact that it only takes a few minutes to go through the entire tapping protocol, some few extra rounds are insignificant in comparison with the benefit of clearing traumatic events that have caused much suffering and have prevented you from expressing your full potential.

"To learn how to forget is more a joy than an art."

Baltazar Gracian

"Memory is like a worker who endeavors to establish a lasting foundation amid the waves."

Marcel Proust.

5.

Planning a Successful EFT Treatment

General Considerations

To apply an EFT treatment is extremely simple. First, you need to contact the emotion that you want to eliminate by tuning your thoughts to the feeling associated with the memory that caused the negative emotion. This is a fundamental step in obtaining the benefit you are seeking from this technique. It is important to be very specific. Do not consider the emotions you want to eliminate in general terms, which is a very common mistake people make when they start using EFT. For instance, *"I am frightened by people with power," "I am not an intelligent person," "My parents always looked down on me."* These are too general. All of these emotions were built upon specific events and those events are the ones that must be addressed to eliminate the underlying negative emotion. To be effective, the general statement *"I am frightened by people with power"* has to be broken down into specific components. Next, you apply EFT treatment to each of the contributing events in order to clear the negative emotion attached to each one.

For instance, a fear of authority figures may be composed of the following specific events:

"My father punished me too severely when I brought home my report card with a C in biology."

"When I was 10 years old, the school principal sent me home when my parents did not pay the school fees."

"My supervisor ridiculed me in front of all the staff in our last month meeting"

As another example, the feeling *"I am afraid of falling into poverty"* is also a general one which can be broken into several contributing elements:

"When I was seven, all of my friends had fashionable toys, but I was so poor I didn't have any."

"When I was twelve, my father lost his job and soon after we received a notice of eviction from our home because we couldn't afford to pay the rent."

"When the factory was acquired, I was laid off and never rehired again."

Each of these events carries an emotional component to the general fear of poverty. Therefore, we need to apply EFT treatments to each of them.

The next step consists in evaluating your emotion using the Subjective Units of Distress scale (SUD). This is a psychological quantitative indicator designed to measure your level of psychological stress; the scale goes from 1 to 10, with 1 being no distress at all and 10 a maximum distress. The number you assign to your distress is an indicator that would let you compare your feelings before and after the treatment, and thus assess your progress.

The next step is to apply the tapping sequences. This involves stimulating with your fingers the meridian end points in a specific order. In the following sections I describe in detail the meridian points locations and their order. At the beginning you will need to follow the points with the book, but the procedure is so simple that you will find it very easy to memorize.

I would like to emphasize that this is the EFT protocol, which is a generalized and simpler procedure derived from the original TFT algorithms. There is a distinction between the TFT and the EFT treatments; I considered both equally effective. However, the TFT tapping sequence varies with each emotion. In other words, there is a specific tapping protocol to address a particular emotion. This results in many different protocols to memorize. On the other hand, there is only one general EFT protocol for all negative emotions. The EFT protocol is very inclusive and does not change according to the emotion. You only need to learn one sequence of tapping points and apply them independently of the negative emotion you want to eradicate. It is based on the principle that by tapping all the meridians ending points, by default you will access the ones that will trigger a relief of the negative emotion. By tapping on all the points you can always be sure you will activate the required ones. Because is a simpler process, the EFT treatment is the focus of this book.

Before introducing the meridian points and tapping sequence, I present the case of one of my clients which illustrates some of the features of EFT treatments previously described: (1) It is extremely effective in clearing deep negative emotions; (2) the client does not need to believe in its effectiveness in order to receive full benefits from its application; (3) its simple application enables the user to do it by himself in a few minutes; and (4) clearing a deep negative emotion usually brings relief to other emotional problems associated with the original issue in the subconscious. This last feature relates to the form in which thoughts and emotions are linked by similarity and association. You will notice that by clearing some specific emotional distress, other negative emotions associated with it will also be cleared without us knowing.

Matthew's Case

This case involves a 37-year-old man that I will call Matthew. He came to see me afflicted with intense stress, insomnia, and upper back muscle spasms so serious that muscle relaxing medication could only temporarily alleviate his discomfort. He was confronting some problems at work. He attributed his troubles to the stress at work, but after doing some taping the emotional discomfort remained almost unchanged.

After some deeper exploration of the events that were going on in his life, we were able to unveil the core of his emotional distress. The main trigger was an upcoming family reunion. He had managed to avoid taking part in family gatherings for eight years with excuses of one sort or another, but this time he had no alternative; the entire family decided to travel to his place of residence to see him. They rented a beach home for a week to have enough time to enjoy each other's company. The thought of being with his mother and brothers made Matthew very anxious. He perceives his mother as a person that complains about everything and demands constant attention; his brothers physically and verbally abused him as a child, an adolescent, and all through his early adulthood. His mother lives in Australia and was getting to an advanced age. Every week when Matthew talks to her on the phone, she ends the conversation saying that the thing she wants the most is to see all of her children in harmony and that she does not want to die knowing that there was not peace in her family.

Matthew felt that this upcoming reunion could be the last time he could see his mother alive. In the past he tried to make peace with his brothers. After extensive psychotherapy he was able to communicate with them again, but the entire family has not been under the same roof since Matthew left for college many years ago. The short brief encounters that they have had always culminated in arguments that brought back issues from the past. Matthew wanted to experiment with EFT because he had read of the effectiveness of this technique in treating anxiety and the positive results that had been obtained in a short period of time. He was also very impressed with the fact that he could continue using the technique on his own for other issues.

In the beginning he was reluctant to believe that the technique could help him with his anxiety. I clearly stated that he did not have to believe in the effectiveness of EFT to receive its benefits. However, from the very beginning, with four complete rounds of EFT treatments his anxiety level decreased from 8 to 3. This case took several sessions because when his anxiety decreased other feelings associated with his family situation reemerged. Pictures of different situations came to his mind. He felt angry toward his mother for not protecting him against the abuses of his father and brothers. He felt rage, embarrassment, and deep sadness. There was a series of complex emotions he thought he had overcome.

It often happens with EFT that after one has cleared the negative energy associated with one particular situation other emotions, directly or indirectly associated with the same incident tend to emerge. A simple analogy between our emotional issues and the peeling of an onion has been used by EFT practitioners to illustrate what takes place when we uncover layer after layer of negative emotions. As you uncover one layer you find many more layers until you get to the point were they are all eliminated. The most important issues to treat are those that keep reoccurring or resurfacing every time when there is a situation that triggers them. The user should carefully examine his or her habits when looking for those core issues. For instance if you get angry each time someone disagrees with your opinion, or if you have an unusual fear of public speaking, chances are they represent core issues of the personality which should be treated. These core issues are considered very valuable; they serve as indicators of unresolved situations which are charged with negative emotion that need to be released. Many times, after treating a traumatic event with EFT, other traumatic events and/or physical discomfort associated with the mayor trauma are also eliminated. When this happens, we wonder why we no longer react the same way we use to when confronted with a situation that in the past, was enough to make us lose control over our emotions.

After the trip, when Matthew returned for his next appointment, he reported that during the week he stayed with his family, he not even once thought of engaging in an argument with his brothers. He did not feel close to them but he was relaxed and surprisingly calmed. He did not feel the need to escape as he always did. He said that they had "civilized conversations." He was also surprised that he found himself lovingly interacting with his mother. He listened to all of her complaints without feeling angry. The memory of the abuses is still with him, but Matthew does not feel the anger and resentment that tormented him before. He stated that he has found forgiveness in his heart.

When Matthew cleared his emotional issues, the physical pain was also alleviated. One of my regular clients recently reported that he had been using EFT for his anxiety because he felt intimidated by his supervisor. After he had worked on issues of self-respect and victimization, the most unusual thing happened to him. He also used to feel so irritated by one of his coworkers; he described him as "the one who knows everything," constantly interrupting everyone and imposing his opinion over that of others. After my client cleared the original issue with his supervisor, he no longer felt upset by his coworker's domineering behavior. When his coworker raises his voice and interrupts anyone, my client now feels sympathy for how much attention this person needs, but no negative emotion.

"And that is how we waste our life: the past becomes like a barrier, it traps you, it locks you into something it no longer exists. You are left stagnant in the dead. And the more experience, more maturity you have, the layers of dead experiences will become thicker around you. You isolate yourself more and more, little by little all the windows are closed. You exist, but alienated, displaced. You are not in communion with life."

Osho.

6.

Procedure for Applying an EFT Treatment

It is Always Available: It is in Your Hands!

PREPARING TO APPLY AN EFT TREATMENT

To apply an EFT treatment is extremely simple, but it requires a very precise set of steps which I describe below. In the following I summarize the basic procedure, which should be sufficient for many self treatments. For more information on TFT or EFT, please visit the corresponding Internet sites (see the section on resources). They contain valuable advice and new techniques developed by many users around the globe. Some users specialize on different areas of EFT applications such as prosperity issues, alcoholism, insomnia, positive thinking, etc.

Deciding on a Negative Emotion to Treat

The first step in applying an EFT treatment is to decide on a negative emotion you want to clear by contacting the memory of the negative emotion. Focus on a specific situation attached to the emotion and be very concrete. Do you feel uneasy about an upcoming meeting? Do you feel nervous about a presentation or a report? Are you angry at someone, or about something? Do you feel sad each time you see someone? Trust your feelings and intuition. If something or someone makes you feel uncomfortable or uneasy, it is because you have unresolved issues with negative emotions attached to them. Those issues should be explored.

Once you have decided to work on a particular negative emotion, you need to rate its intensity. You do this on a scale from 1 to 10, with 1 being almost no intensity and 10 extremely intense. This is a subjective measure of the degree of distress. It is important to rate this intensity in order to assess the effectiveness of the treatment once it has been applied.

Tunning to Your Emotion

Once you have decided what to work on, you then apply the treatment while consciously tunning your thoughts to that specific negative emotion. This requires a conscious effort to remember a stressful situation that brings negative feelings. Maintain your concentration on the feeling throughout the entire treatment.

For example, say you feel nervous about an upcoming interview or public speaking engagement and you wish to clear this feeling so as to enhance your performance. Hence, during the two or so minutes spent in the treatment you need to concentrate on your feelings of insecurity and nervousness. This is done by imagining that you are in the interview or at the podium speaking and allowing yourself to feel stressed and nervous. Thus, while tapping with your fingers on the meridian end points you imagine the stressful event *and feel* the negative emotion.

If you want to work on a negative emotion attached to an event that occurred in the past, then you need to remember the past event at its critical point. For example, if you want to clear the anger related to an incident when you were assaulted verbally or physically you will have to remember the incident as it happened to you while tapping on the meridian end points. This may be difficult as it may bring back intense memories of the event, but you do not have to go all the way to the bottom of the emotion. You need to tune into the emotion, but not re-live all the pain in its profundity. If while tunning to the negative emotion, you feel like breathing deeply, or shaking, feel free to do so. The discharge of energy may be expressed in any way you feel like.

It is important to emphasize that for the emotion to be cleared the treatment must be very specific. In other words, if you wish to eliminate some anger you experience towards a person, you need to isolate this emotion from other attached emotions you may feel towards this person. This is especially important if the person in question has a long history of events dealing with you. In other words, if you feel uncomfortable in the presence of a colleague or a relative, the uncomfortable feelings may be composed of different feelings. For instance, anger due to an event in the distant past, sadness because of your disapproval of this person's behavior towards others, and attraction because you may feel intrigued about certain aspects of his personality. These are feelings attached in layers and stored in the unconscious mind in complex ways. Thus, what you need to do is apply an EFT treatment for each specific event and clear each of those emotions. For instance, apply a treatment to clear the anger. Repeat until you get a rating of 1. Next apply another treatment to an important event that caused you to disapprove the person's behavior and thus clear the feeling of sadness. Next you apply another treatment in which you would focus on an event or a feature you remember that caused you to feel intrigued. This process is followed until all feelings of uneasiness towards this person are cleared. Remember that each treatment should be repeated until a rating of 1 is reached.

Select an Appropriate Affirmation

While tunning to the specific emotion to be cleared and while tapping the meridian end points, a verbal affirmation should be repeated. One popular one is the following:

"I deeply and completely accept myself, even though I have this (problem, feeling, of fear, guilt, anger, etc.)."

Some EFT practitioners recommend to select a positive affirmation that emphasizes overcoming the negative feeling. The following are examples:

"Even though I feel nervous about this presentation, I hereby decide to be calm and relaxed."

"Even though I am angry at John, I hereby forgive him and decide to be at peace with myself."

"Even though I feel very sad about what happened last night, I decide to let it go and be happy."

"Even though I am ashamed of what I did, I ask for forgiveness and I forgive myself."

"Even though I feel afraid of applying for this promotion, I trust myself and decide to be calm and relaxed."

"Even though you (name of person) hurt me when I was little, I forgive you, I wish you the best, and I let you go."

These affirmations have two components: First, they acknowledge the negative feeling, and second they offer a phrase of empowerment, a resolution to overcome the problem.

Remember the unconscious mind is susceptible of verbal suggestion. A carefully selected positive affirmation is very effective when repeated in conjunction with the mental attuning to the specific feeling, while you are doing physical stimulation (i.e., the tapping).

To develop the phrase, use common sense. Build a phrase that would address the problem. To do this, ask yourself what the problem is, and the answer you obtain is the focal point of the setup phrase.

Physical Stimulation: Tapping the Meridian End Points

Each EFT treatment contains a series of tapping maneuvers on certain points on the body. These points constitute the terminal skin locations of energy meridians in the body. The stimulation of these points goes to the exact location of the emotional distress stored in the unconscious mind. The location of the thought field associated with the emotional distress is found by tunning with the negative feeling. The stimulation causes the discharge of the energy associated with the negative emotion and thus restores the natural flow of energy. The stimulation is done by tapping the points with your fingers. You use the index and middle fingers of either hand. Tapping with the two fingers cover a larger area than that of the end point and you do not need to concentrate so much on its exact location. Tap solidly, but not too hard so as to hurt yourself. Tap approximately 10 times on each point, but do not worry about counting. The frequency or speed of tapping is up to you. You can tap repeatedly with your finger tips, but you should find the frequency that you are comfortable with.

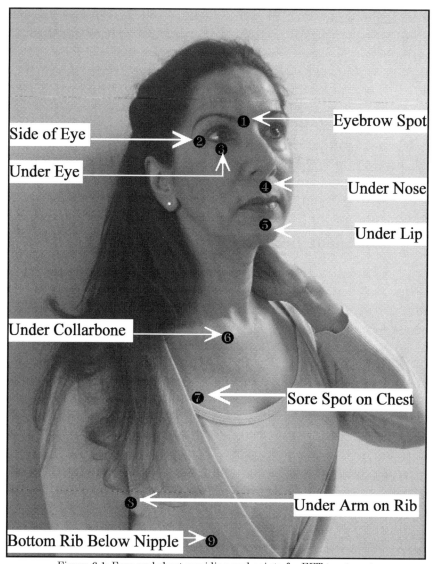

Figure 6.1: Face and chest meridian end points for EFT treatment

There are 15 meridian end points used in EFT. A treatment consists in tapping on each of these points sequentially. Study the description below and Figures 6.1, 6.2, and 6.3 to memorize their location. The points are located on either side of the body. In other words, each point on the right side of the face, chest, or hand has a counterpart on the left side respectively. You can tap on either side or if you prefer you can tap on both sides at the same time by using both hands.

The following is a description of the points. When memorizing them, remember that the numbers have been assigned in sequence from the head down. The numbers refer to those on Figures 6.1, 6.2, and 6.3:

1.   *Bridge of Nose by Eyebrow*. At the beginning of the eyebrow, just above and to one side of the nose (Figure 6.1).

2.   *Side of Eye*. On the bone bordering the outside corner of the eye (Figure 6.1).

3.   *Under Eye*. On the bone under an eye about 1 inch below the eyeball (Figure 6.1).

4.   *Under Nose*. On the small area between the bottom of the nose and the upper lip (Figure 6.1).

5.   *Under Mouth*. Midway between the point of the chin and the bottom of the lower lip (Figure 6.1).

6.   *Under Collar Bone*. The junction where the sternum (breastbone), collarbone and the first rib meet. To locate it, first place your finger on the U-shaped notch at the top of the breastbone (i.e., the place where a man knots his tie). From the bottom of the U move the forefinger down toward the navel 1 inch and then go to the left (or right) 1 inch (Figure 6.1).

7.   *Sore Spot on Chest*. This is the spot where lymphatic congestion occurs sometimes. To locate it, first place your

finger on the U-shaped notch at the top of the breastbone (i.e., the place where a man knots his tie). From the bottom of the U move the forefinger down toward the navel 3 inches and then go to the left (or right) 3 inches (Figure 6.1).

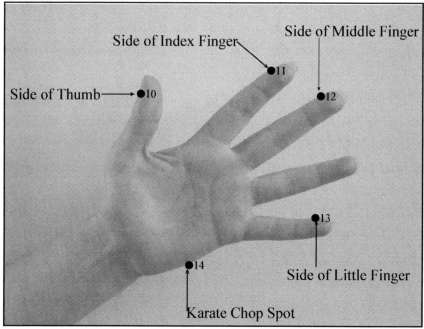

Figure 6.2: Hand meridian end points for EFT treatment

8.   *Under Arm on Rib*. On the side of the body at a point even with the nipple (for men) or in the middle of the bra strap (for women). It is located about 4 inches below the arm pit (Figure 6.1).

9.   *Bottom Rib Below Nipple*. One inch below the nipple (for men). For women, tap under the breast, where the skin of the breast meets the chest wall (Figure 6.1).

10.   *Side of Thumb*. On the outside edge of the thumb at a point even with the base of the thumbnail (Figure 6.2).

11.   *Side of Index Finger*. On the side of the index finger (the side facing the thumb) at a point even with the base of the finger nail (Figure 6.2).

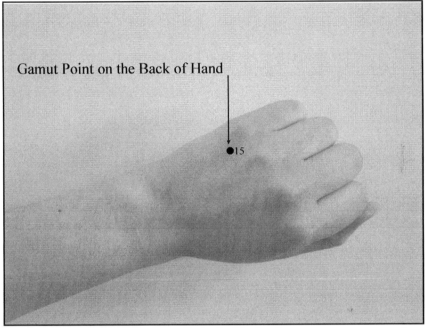

Figure 6.3: Gamut point on the back of the hand

12.   *Side of Middle Finger*. On the side of the middle finger (the side closest to the thumb) at a point even with the base of the fingernail (Figure 6.2).

13.   *Side of Little Finger*. On the side of the little finger (the side closest to the thumb) at a point even with the base of the fingernail (Figure 6.2).

14.   *Karate Chop Spot*. In the middle of the fleshy part on the outside of the hand between the top of the wrist bone and the base of the little finger (Figure 6.2).

15. *The Gamut Point*. On the back of the hand, between the bones of the ring finger and the little finger, half an inch below the knuckles (Figure 6.3).

Sequence of Tapping the Points

The sequence and order of tapping the meridian end points is the following:

❐ First, tap the karate chopping point number 14.
❐ Next, tap the bridge of nose point number 1.
❐ Next, tap the side of eye point number 2.
❐ Next, tap under the eye point number 3.
❐ Next, tap under the nose point number 4.
❐ Next, tap under mouth point number 5.
❐ Next, tap under collarbone point number 6.
❐ Next, tap the sore spot on chest point number 7.
❐ Next, tap under the arm on rib point number 8.
❐ Next, tap on bottom rib below nipple point number 9.
❐ Next, tap on side of thumb point number 10.
❐ Next, tap side of index finger point number 11.
❐ Next, tap side of middle finger point number 12.
❐ Next, tap side of little finger point number 13.

❐ Next, tap the Gamut point number 15 while performing the following sequence:

   ■ Close your eyes for about 2 seconds (if they were open).
   ■ Open your eyes for about 2 seconds.
   ■ Close your eyes for 2 seconds.
   ■ Open your eyes and look down to one side for about

2 seconds.

- Look down to the other side for 2 seconds.
- Roll eyes in a circle in one direction for about 2 seconds.
- Roll eyes in the opposite direction for about 2 seconds.
- Hum a tune for about 2 seconds (a portion of any song you like, e.g. "Happy Birthday").
- In a low voice count slowly from 1 to 5.
- Again hum a tune for about 2 seconds.

❐ Repeat the tapping sequence: tap again point 14 and then each of points 1 through 13 as described above

The eye movements as well as the humming and counting procedures were discovered by Dr. Roger Callahan as stimulating to different parts of the brain. He stated that the humming and counting stimulated the right and left sides of the brain, respectively. Theoretically the right side of the brain becomes receptive to the treatment as it is activated by humming and the tapping of the gamut point. The same occurs for the left side of the brain due to the counting and tapping. As for the eye movements, Callahan found that each movement accessed different areas of the brain. All of these procedures combined ensure that the entire brain is made receptive to the treatment.

Summary of Tapping Sequence

Begin tapping point 14 (karate chop point), then each of the points from 1 through 13. Then go on to point 15 while doing the eyes and humming exercise. Next, tap again point 14, followed by each of the points 1 through 13. This completes one full treatment. It should be noted that point 15 along with the humming, eye movement and counting is only done at the end of the first round.

Effects of EFT Treatments

EFT treatments have no negative side effects and will not interfere with any other form of therapy you may be receiving. The whole tapping sequence should take you about a couple of minutes to complete. You may tap on either the left or right side points. You may notice the release of energy out of some of the points in the form of a tingling sensation. It is important that you drink water prior to and after the treatments. Increased thirst is a side effect of applying EFT treatments. The feeling of thirst implies the consumption of water by the process of energy release. Most people report increased feelings of peace and relaxation after any treatment.

You may also notice a reduction in the degree of intensity of the negative emotion as you progress with the sequence. It is important to complete the entire treatment even if you feel completely relieved. Once you finish a treatment, you need to rate again the intensity of the negative emotion on the same subjective scale from 1 to 10. It is common to obtain a drastic reduction with just one treatment. For long-term chronic emotions, several treatments may be necessary. Repeat the treatment until the emotion has been reduced to a rating of 1.

It is also important to keep your focus on the specific emotion throughout the entire sequence. This cannot be sufficiently stressed because the success of the treatment depends on this. As you progress through the tapping, the reduction of the intensity of the emotion usually brings up other related negative emotions stored in the subconscious mind. It is recommended that you keep a mental focus on the original one and finish the entire treatment until it is reduced to a rating of 1. Then, do a complete sequence on the other related issue that may have come up during the treatment. Keeping a notebook with your observations will help you plan your treatments. As you work on a given issue, other related issues will surface. These related issues are stored in your subconscious mind shadowed by the higher intensity of the original problem. In between sequences, take note of these secondary issues.

For example, imagine you are tapping to clear your anger towards a given person. You tune into your feelings of anger by remembering and replaying an argument you had with this person. While doing so, you may remember all of a sudden an unrelated incident when your father punished you when you where very little. Thus, what you need to do is to keep tapping while mentally focusing on the anger feelings towards the first person and finish the original treatment until it has decreased to 1. In your notebook write the incident with your father that surfaced during the treatment and proceed to do a complete round of tapping on the latter until it has come to 1.

I recommend reserving a few minutes every day to apply treatments on the issues that emerge in your mind, either triggered by external situations you face at the present time, or that surface during the treatment of other issues. I suggest taking one hour or so of your time to sit quietly and write the events and issues that in the past caused you distress. Be as thorough as possible. Then, go over the list and put an asterisk besides the most important ones (i.e., the most distressful). Begin dedicating a few minutes every day to treat each of the important ones. You will notice that by clearing some of the most distressful events in your life, the other issues that you thought were also important suddenly become just memories without much to them.

By systematically clearing the various layers of our negative emotions, we gradually become free of our complexes and distressful memories. In essence, we open opportunities for a happier and more meaningful life, one that is free from automatic, irrational and painful reactions.

Other "side effects" of clearing your negative emotions include physical reactions. It has been reported that many physical ailments improve after we clear negative emotions which are seemingly unrelated to the physical problem. These include migraine headaches, allergies, arthritis, back pain, vision problems, digestive anomalies, and even more chronic physical diseases. The association between mind and body has been known since ancient times, and only recently has main stream science begun to recognize it. Many chronic diseases are the result of energy imbalances in our emotions. Be attentive and observe your habits, your attitudes towards work and life, and treat any negative feelings about them. Investigate each chronic pain or a physical problem you have and see if there is an emotional issue behind it. A good way of doing it is by applying an EFT treatment to the pain and observing what feelings come up during the sequence. Always trust your intuition when it comes to following the feelings that come up during EFT treatments. Perfect health is our natural right and the result of a balance between mind and body.

When you clear a chronic pattern, or a series of many issues during a session, some temporary emotional or physical discomfort could occur. You may feel sad or experience pain in the chest or stomach. A client worked for several days on some long-term chronic feelings from his childhood. In the following days he began to feel what could be described as a strong pain in his stomach near the solar plexus. It was as if he had indigestion with an accompanied bloated stomach, except that it was not related to diet and it did not disappear for several days, regardless of what he ate. Upon further exploring his feelings, he discovered that unconsciously he did not really want to give up some of his negative patterns. These distressful patterns caused him much animosity and pain for many years. However, these patterns were also a defense mechanism learned and developed to protect him after certain traumatic events in his childhood. They were a "solution"–however inappropriate–to deal with a hostile world.

Some of your own patterns may have a similar resistance. You may feel afraid to face the world without the pattern. Many people do not really want to be cured from their chronic emotional or physical diseases, especially if the disease brings some form of "reward." Some people receive compensation for their diagnosed disability. They may feel unconsciously afraid to give up what has become a form of life and face the uncertainty of having to work again with a healthy body. The reward for a disease is not always monetary. Some people get much attention, compassion, and special treatment while suffering from a disease. They may not want to give that up. Of course this resistance to heal is unconscious. It will have to be discovered hidden behind the pattern and may surface in one way or another during your conscious attempts to clear the pattern. For severe chronic patterns the skills of a trained EFT counselor will be necessary in discovering and treating the core issues.

ALL IN ALL: THE ESSENTIAL STEPS FOR APPLYING AN EFT TREATMENT

The following exercise summarizes the steps on the

application of an EFT treatment. You should have carefully read the above sections prior to the treatment and familiarized yourself with the locations of each of the points.

Exercise 6.1: Applying an EFT Treatment

Objective

To clear any negative feelings, complexes, fixations, or undesirable patterns. These include: fear; self doubt; anxiety; grief over a loss of a loved one; anger; negative memories involving rape or assault; fear of sports or public performances; phobias; tobacco, alcohol or drug dependency; panic attacks; post traumatic stress disorders; depression; insomnia, etc.

Description

First, decide which specific emotion or problem you want to clear. I remark that the emotion or event must be very specific. The emotion may be a past event, as in the memory of a traumatic incident or argument, or it could be in the future as in the fear of an upcoming public or social event. Decide on a mental picture to play in your imagination during the treatment. This could be recalling portions of the past event or imagining the future situations. Rate the emotion with a subjective scale from 1 to 10, with 1 being minimal distress, and 10 being maximum. Also, decide on an affirmation that (1) acknowledges the negative feeling, and (2) offers a statement of freedom from the problem.

Next, close your eyes if possible, and tune into the specific emotion. In other words, replay in your imagination the distressful event or memory and allow your self to feel the negative emotion (fear, anger, sadness, etc.).

While tuning into your emotion, repeat your affirmation verbally if possible, or mentally. For example,

"Even though I feel (emotion, memory), I hereby decide to be (opposite emotion, freedom from memory)."

While mentally tunning to your emotion and verbally repeating the affirmation, tap with your index and middle fingers of either hand each of the meridian end points about 10 times. Do not be concerned with counting. Begin tapping point 14 (karate chop point), then each of points 1 through 13, and then point 15 while doing the eyes and humming exercise (Figures 6.1, 6.2, 6.3 and related explanations). Next, tap again point 14, followed by each of the points 1 through 13. The location of the points and the order of tapping must be memorized prior to the treatment, or have this book close by for reference.

Possible Results

When the treatment is finished, rate again the intensity of the emotion from 1 to 10. Most treatments result in a significant reduction in the intensity of the emotion. If it has not come down significantly, repeat the treatment. If after two or three treatments, the emotion has a low rating but does not disappear, the situation may not be specific enough, or there is resistance to heal, or the emotion is linked to other physical or emotional issues that must be addressed. In Chapter 7 we will discuss these problems. Watch for the emotions or feelings that surface while doing the treatment. These are good clues to follow up with future treatments. However, you should finish the treatment with the original emotion. Write your impressions in your notebook as soon as possible. The "interfering" emotions that emerge during a treatment are valuable pieces of information that will soon be forgotten or repressed in memory if you do not record them.

Summary

The following are the quick steps for this exercise. The treatment itself consists of the simultaneous tuning with the negative emotion, the repetition of the affirmation, and the tapping of the points in the precise sequence.

1. *Decide on a Negative Emotion to Clear*. Choose a negative emotion attached to a specific situation to work and rate its intensity from 1 to 10. Select a mental picture or memory to recall during treatment. Decide on an affirmation to repeat during the treatment.

2. *Tune into the Specific Emotion*. Close your eyes, remember the distressful event and play it in your imagination all during the entire treatment. Feel the negative emotion.

3. *Repeat the Affirmation*. While tuning into your emotion, verbally repeat the affirmation. After you setup your complete phrase while tapping the karate chop point, you may use a shortened, reminder phrase for the rest of the treatment.

4. *Tap the Meridian End Points*. While tunning into your emotion, and repeating the affirmation, tap with your

fingers about 10 times on each point in the following order: begin tapping point 14 (karate chop point), then each of points 1 through 13, and then point 15 while doing the eyes and humming exercise (Figures 6.1, 6.2, 6.3 and related explanations). Next, tap again point 14, followed by each of the points 1 through 13.

5. ***Rate the Emotion***. After the treatment, rate again the intensity of the negative emotion. If it has not come down to 1, repeat the treatment.

Note: Steps 2, 3, and 4 are done simultaneously throughout the treatment

Table 6.1: Correspondences Between EFT Points and Emotions

Point	Associated Emotion
1. Eyebrow spot	Trauma, frustration
2. Side of eye	Rage, bad mood
3. Under eye	Anxiety, addiction, phobia, fear
4. Under nose	Embarrassment, shame, depression, nervousness, anxiety, fear, guilt
5. Under mouth	Shame
6. Collarbone	Depression, obsession
7. Sore spot on chest	Sadness, depression
9. Under arm	Fear
10. Thumb	Disdain, impatience, prejudice, anger
11. Index finger	Guilt, remorse, shame, regret
12. Middle finger	Headache, worries
13. Little finger	Anger
14. Karate chop	Sadness, anguish, grief, remorse
15. Gamut point	Depression, physical pain

RELATIONSHIP BETWEEN EFT POINTS AND EMOTIONS TREATED

The following table (Table 6.1) illustrates the correspondences between the EFT meridian end points and emotions treated by their stimulation. This should serve as a guide to prepare a treatment that addresses a specific emotion. By emphasizing stimulation of the corresponding point you can maximize the effectiveness of treatments. I recommend you use your intuition when running a treatment. If you feel that a given point is more sensitive or is relieving you more than the others, then try to stimulate that one longer.

SHORT VERSION OF THE EFT TREATMENT

Gary Craig has developed an EFT short version. You may be asking yourself a valid question. Why do I need a shorter version of EFT when the entire procedure only takes a few minutes? Although the entire EFT technique is always preferable to the shortcuts, there are instances in which the shortcuts are very convenient and equally effective:

1.   If you are in public and you do not want to attract attention. For instance, if you are in a meeting where some issues make you uncomfortable. Take a short break, apply a short treatment, and come back feeling better and in total control.

2.   If you are helping another person or if you are a therapist working with several clients, the time that you save is very valuable.

The following is the shortcut tapping sequence. The numbers correspond to the point numbers as illustrated in Figures 6.1 and 6.3.

❏ *Bridge of Nose by Eyebrow (point 1)*. At the beginning of the eyebrow, just above and to one side of the nose (Figure 6.1).

❏ *Side of Eye (point 2)*. On the bone bordering the outside corner of the eye (Figure 6.1).

❏ *Under Eye (point 3)*. On the bone under an eye about 1 inch below the pupil (Figure 6.1).

❏ *Under Nose (point 4)*. On the small area between the bottom of the nose and the top of the upper lip (Figure 6.1).

❏ *Under Mouth (point 5)*. Midway between the point of the chin and the bottom of the lower lip (Figure 6.1).

❏ *Under Collar Bone (point 6)*. The junction where the sternum (breastbone), collarbone and the first rib meet. To locate it, first place your finger on the U-shaped notch at the top of the breastbone (i.e., the place where a man knots his tie). From the bottom of the U move the forefinger down toward the navel 1 inch and then go to the left (or right) 1 inch (Figure 6.1).

❏ *Under Arm on Rib (point 7)*. On the side of the body at a point even with the nipple (for men) or in the middle of the bra strap (for women). It is located about 4 inches below the arm pit (Figure 6.1).

❏ *The Gamut Point (point 15)*. On the back of the hand, half an inch behind the mid point between the knuckles at the base of the ring finger and the little finger (Figure 6.3). Tap this point while performing following the floor-to-ceiling eye roll routine:

- Holding your head straight, move your eyes down to look at the floor.
- Move your eyes slowly upward to the ceiling.

This eye-roll routine step could take the emotion you are working from a low of 2 to 1, eliminating the need for another round of the basic sequence.

7.

EFT Special Techniques

Dealing With Special Problems and Improving Treatment Effectiveness

In the last chapter we described the basic technique for applying an EFT treatment, along with its short-cut variant. This chapter discusses some of the problems that may be encountered when applying treatments and the procedure to overcome them. In particular, we discuss the case of psychological reversal, which is behind many deeply ingrained or chronic distress patterns, and also in situations when the method appears not to work. In this chapter there are also some techniques that will improve EFT effectiveness. These techniques have been proven to be very useful in treating a wide range of emotional problems by EFT specialists and the public in general.

WHEN EFT SEEMS INEFFECTIVE: PSYCHOLOGICAL REVERSAL (RESISTANCE TO CHANGE)

Sometimes an EFT treatment appears to be ineffective in spite of our careful efforts <u>and persistence</u> to apply it correctly. This situation occurs commonly when attempting to clear deep patterns of behavior or long-term additions. Some people consciously want to liberate themselves form their crippling emotional distress but at their unconscious level they do not want to let go of their fears or addictions. These negative and distressful feelings serve a purpose in their life and keep them "safe" by maintaining the type of life and behavior that are well known to them. If they let go of their pattern, they will have to learn to act in a different way unknown to them. Confronting unknown feelings frighten us. Although this process may sound like a contradictory statement, this is a way of protection that some people develop without being aware of it. In many cases, a disease or disability may have real benefits to the person. For instance, a person may receive monetary compensation, compassion from others, or special treatment thanks to a debilitating or crippling condition. In these cases, the patient may be unconsciously reluctant to be healed. This may imply having to let go of any rewards and learning a new trade or new behavior. Without treating psychological reversal, EFT treatments would have limited effectiveness in these situations. Callahan calls this apparent self-sabotage to change Psychological Reversal.

Psychological Reversal is more common that we care to admit. We set clear goals in our life, such as: getting a new job; to stop smoking; to lose weigh; to make more money; to stop drinking; to get a new contract; or stop consuming drugs. Sometimes it happens that even when we consciously know we want to accomplish these goals we do not take the necessary steps, but contrary to that, we continue doing the things that are damaging to us. This is because of our internal resistance to change. Negative thinking and self-defeating thoughts are to blame for this condition.

For EFT treatments to work, Psychological Reversal has to be corrected. Callahan attributes the existence of Psychological Reversal to a reversal of polarity in the body's energy system, the internal energy flow becomes inverted or blocked. How do we correct Psychological Reversal? By tapping on the Karate Chop point (see Figure 7.1) to break the energy flow obstruction. If you apply an EFT treatment and notice that the condition you are treating does not change, consider the presence of Psychological Reversal. Your best indicator is to evaluate your discomfort or distress level by using the measuring scale that was previously described. If you notice no change or improvement in the condition you are treating, then you have reason to suspect the presence of Psychological Reversal. In those cases you have to apply a correction for such a condition.

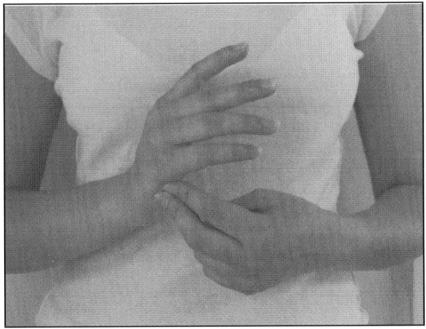

Figure 7.1: the Karate Chop Point.

VARIATIONS ON THE STATEMENT PHRASE

In the original EFT procedure developed by Gary Craig, the affirmation phrase was divided in two parts: a "setup phrase," which is a sentence that acknowledges the negative emotion, and a short version of it, or the "reminder phrase," which summarizes the setup phrase with a couple or words. The setup phrase is to be repeated about three times at the beginning of the treatment while tapping point 14 (the karate chop point), or point 7 (the chest sore point). The reminder phrase, is to be repeated while tapping the rest of the points. The reminder phrase keeps you focused on the emotion being treated. The general setup phrase proposed by Craig is:

"Even though I have this (feeling, negative emotion), I completely love and accept myself."

For instance, when treating a feeling of fear about driving for the first time in a rented car in Paris during an upcoming vacation a client stated his setup phrase as follows:

"Even though I am afraid of driving in Paris, a city I have never been to, in a car I have never driven, I totally and completely love and accept myself."

This phrase was repeated while tapping point 14 (the karate chop point), or point 7 (the chest sore point). Now, the short reminder phrase in this case was:

"Fear of driving in Paris."

This short summary phrase was repeated while tapping the rest of the treatment points. The reminder phrase is easy to memorize without distracting from the emotion, which is essential to the treatment.

One of the drawbacks of the traditional setup-reminder phrase is that it puts too much emphasis on the negative emotion, rather than in the positive re-emergence from it. In the case above, the sentence *"fear of driving"* emphasizes on the negative feeling, rather than on the positive (e.g., *"I drive confidently"*). For these reasons, in chapter 6 we introduced a general phrase that (1) acknowledged the negative emotion and (2) offered a positive statement to overcome it.

DIFFICULTY FOCUSING ON AN EMOTION

If during an EFT treatment you find yourself having difficulties focusing on the emotional problem or contacting your feelings Gary Craig recommends creating in your mind an image of the problem and to be very attentive of any physical sensation you may feel. While thinking about the problem, be aware of any tension, discomfort, ache, or pain in your body. Concentrate your attention on that physical sensation and apply the EFT technique by tapping at each point. Pay particular attention to any negative thought that may emerge and tap on it until you feel that nothing else is surfacing into your conscious mind. Remember that one particular event may have many ramifications. It would be necessary to work diligently to clear all of the negative emotions associated with the problem to facilitate the healing process.

Tap on any issue that may emerge. Sometimes it happens that you may think that a random thought that just "happened to emerge" into your conscious mind is totally unrelated or insignificant to any of the emotions you are clearing at that time, but the fact remains that if it surfaced into your conscious mind it is because that thought has some significance. Do not be judgmental, trust your feelings, and take that emerging thought seriously. It is advisable to consider that thought and to tap on the issue. It may lead you to something else and help you to clear some emotional issues that otherwise you may have overlooked.

RELATIONSHIP BETWEEN PHYSICAL PROBLEMS AND NEGATIVE EMOTIONS

As described in the previous section, a negative emotion may be attached to other seemingly unrelated problems. It is often reported that the related problem is physical in nature. You may think that the physical discomfort you may be experiencing at the time is not associated with your emotions, but there is a strong correlation between our negative emotion and physical pain. Many physical problems have an emotional foundation. The neck, back, legs, and arms are especially sensitive parts that store not only stress and tension but also more chronic dysfunctions.

The EFT Internet site (www.emofree.com) reports the experiences of many practitioners who found that by treating and relieving negative emotions the clients also found an unexpected connection to seemingly unrelated physical problems. They have also found that when a client complains about chronic physical pain, a subsequent EFT treatment uncovers the fact that the pain had an emotional foundation. However, some people have difficulties understanding this relationship, particularly when they think that the symptoms they are experiencing seem to be caused "entirely" by a physical injury.

For instance, Stephanie Wood, a Canadian EFT practitioner had a client who complained about shoulder pain. The client was convinced that it was due to a physical injury. First, Wood used EFT to address the physical pain only. Then, several treatments were done during which the client was asked to repeat the following setup phrase. These sentences acknowledged the physical pain and opened the mind for any information as to its cause:

"Even though I have this shoulder pain and I don't know what is causing it, I love and accept myself."

"Even though I might have this shoulder pain for a reason but I don't know what that is, I love and accept myself."

"Even though this shoulder pain might have some information for me, I choose to acknowledge this and hear it on some level, consciously or subconsciously."

"Even though I may have needed this shoulder pain in the past, I am now ready to let it go, I love and accept myself."

"Even though this shoulder pain has served some purpose, I choose to now know this on some level, consciously or subconsciously."

"Even though I have this stupid shoulder pain, I forgive myself and anyone else who may have contributed to this pain."

Wood reported that affirmations such as the last one are very useful to unveil new directions for the client. She also recommends the use of humor as a positive element to change the clients' perception about the nature of their affliction. While tapping the points, she reported the use of the following reminder phrases which can be substituted by any other physical discomfort:

"This shoulder pain."

"It's telling me something."

"It has served a purpose."

"I don't know what it is."

"I don't need to know."

"It's OK not to know."

"I'm ready to let it all go"

"It's served a purpose."

"And now I can move on."

"I don't need to take this out on my body anymore."

"Everything that is in my shoulder."

"Everything that it means."

"I honor it and let it go."

This process brings old memories that the client had not connected with the current injury. Once the memories and old emotions emerge in your conscious mind you can eliminate them through EFT. Once you have discovered the core of the problem, it only needs your persistence to be free from it.

ASPECTS OF MULTIPLICITY IN EFT TREATMENTS

In many instances you only need to apply a few rounds of EFT treatment to get complete emotional release, but there are some occasions in which you apply the EFT treatment and you notice that the intensity has not decreased even after you have applied the treatment several times. At this point you start to wonder if you are doing something wrong or if EFT does not apply to your case. Do not despair. It is possible that the issue you are treating has many ramifications, each with its own emotional charge, but the essence remains untreated.

For instance, if you have a fear of flying you can apply EFT to *"this fear of flying"* and you will probably feel some benefit out of this, but if you do not notice any changes in your emotions it means that there are some aspects that have to be addressed in order to eradicate the core of this fear. You can ask yourself: *what is it that scares me the most about flying?* The answer that comes to your mind may be *"the time when the plane takes off,"* *"the fear of the altitude,"* *"the loud noise,"* etc. Next, you proceed to tap on each of these aspects of your fear by applying an EFT treatment until you get to 1 on the measurement scale. Then you ask yourself: *"Is there anything else about flying that still frightens me?"* If the answer is yes, imagine that situation that still frightens you while applying as many rounds of EFT as necessary until the fear is totally gone. As a last test, picture yourself flying; you should not feel any negative emotions.

Another point to take into account is the emotional shifting that may occur while applying EFT treatments. For instance, you may be working on a feeling of rejection. While applying the treatment, you notice the rejection feeling is gone but it has been replaced by one of anxiety. This offers you an opportunity to clear related emotional blockages you probably did not know you had. You should proceed in the same way described above, until the anxiety is gone. In the end, you should be able to remember any previously stressful situation without feeling anything. A past experience is just that, a memory and nothing else.

OTHER TECHNIQUES TO ENHANCE EFT EFFECTIVENESS

The basic tapping points described in Chapter 6 have been used to complement other techniques or methods that further enhance the effectiveness of EFT.

The Choice Method

A method developed by Patricia Carrington can be used at the end of a session after you have cleared important emotional issues. You can finish your session with a relevant "choice," a positive affirmation that consolidates the emotional progress achieved with EFT by reprogramming your subconscious mind. This method was created as an extension of EFT by modifying the default statement with the use of a choice that states desirable behavior.

In the original EFT method, the default statement is:

"Even though I have this problem (you introduce your problem here), *I love and accept myself."*

With this method, you affirm your intention to change while at the same time it puts you in control. It gives you the alternative, the choice to change. For instance, one of my clients who was terrified of public speaking wanted to work on her fear. She had to go to a conference to present a research paper and was very anxious about it. We used EFT to get to the core issue of her fear but in the end she practiced using the Choice Method. She used the following affirmation:

"Even thought I feel very nervous about speaking at this conference, I choose to feel confident and relaxed during my presentation and every time I speak in public."

In the first part of this affirmation the client acknowledges her feelings about public speaking, but finishes her affirmation with a positive decision to be confident and relaxed.

Select the right wording for the choice. This constitutes a

way to obtain help from your subconscious mind which is very powerful and impressionable. When the affirmation is stated in the form of a choice, it is easy to be accepted by your subconscious mind.

Sometimes it happens that the chosen statement does not feel real to you. For instance, the statement *"I feel confident and relaxed when I speak in public"* may not sound or feel right to you. It is as if there is a little voice inside that contradicts the affirmation. You feel you are acting out the statement, but you do not really believe it is true. In those cases the affirmation loses its power. In developing an effective choice statement, follow these guidelines:

Be Specific

Select an affirmation that specifically states what you want to achieve. For instance, if you have a business and you would like to see it growing but you feel uncomfortable promoting it, you could say: *Even though I feel uncomfortable taking the initiative to promote my business, I now choose to make 6 promotional visits per week and I choose to be relaxed, calm, and confident when talking to new potential costumers.* There is no ambiguity in this statement. You clearly state what you want to accomplish. You can notice the difference with this other inadequate affirmation: *Even though I feel uncomfortable taking the initiative to promote my business I now choose to make it grow.*

Be Positive

Always state your affirmation in positive terms. The reason for this is that our unconscious mind only follows direct commands that are deductive in nature. Since we want and need the cooperation of our subconscious mind, always remember that affirmations are orders we give to ourselves and for them to be effective they have to be stated in positive terms.

Here is an example of a positive affirmation developed by a client who had a problem with one of her coworkers:

"Even though I feel anxious when Ellen comes to my office every morning, I now choose to feel relaxed, self-confident and assertive."

Note that it would have been an inappropriate choice to say:

"Even though I feel anxious when Ellen comes to my office every morning, I choose not to feel intimidated by her presence."

The latter is a negative statement not likely to be accepted by the deductive subconscious mind.

Make Decisions that Pertain to You

Make choices and decisions that only pertain to your own feelings because you have no control over other people's lives. Even when it is something positive you want for another person, you risk making an inadequate affirmation when you want to make choices on behalf of others. EFT is a very powerful method to change the way you feel or react in order to build your life the way you envision it, but the focus is on controlling your own feelings, not those of others.

For instance, the following would be an effective

statement:

"Even thought my mother abused me when I was a child, I choose to forgive her."

The phrase gives you the power to change your feelings. On the other hand, the following affirmation would be ineffective:

"I choose to have my mother repent for what she did to me when I was a child."

You have no control over your mother's feelings.

The Movie Technique

The objective of this technique is to assist you in the process of being specific. The effectiveness of EFT is highly magnified when you focus your attention on one concrete event rather than on a general issue. Gary Craig developed this technique to assist clients in distress to be specific and to make the most out of their EFT session. When people feel overwhelmed by their emotions, they tend to talk in general rather than in particular terms. Craig suggests that if you cannot make a mental "movie" of your situation then the problem is too general to be undertaken. For example, *"I have always let people take advantage of me"* represents a very broad problem which is integrated by many situations in which this person lets others take advantage of him. To work effectively with the Movie Technique, the problem will have to be broken down into more detailed events.

When using this technique consider the following guidelines:

The Length of the Movie

Your mental movie should not take days or months to play in your imagination. If you think in terms of days or months, then you are not being specific enough.

The Title of the Movie

Give your movie a title. This will help you narrow down on one particular situation. For instance, *"Lauren Stealing Markers from John and Telling Everyone in the Class That I Did It."*

Rate the Intensity of the Movie

Think about your movie. As you vividly imagine it, evaluate how it makes you feel now, and rate its intensity from 1 to 10.

Apply an EFT Treatment While Playing the Movie

To reduce the intensity of the emotions associated with your movie, apply an EFT treatment while mentally playing your movie in your imagination. Choose a setup phrase related to the title of the movie. For instance, using the example of Lauren stealing the markers, given above, a good setup phrase would be:

"Even though Lauren lied about stealing the markers, I forgive her and forgive myself for not speaking up."

The short reminder phrase for the rest of the treatment should also be taken from the title of the movie. For instance, in the same example about the markers a good reminder phrase would be:

"I forgive Lauren, I forgive myself."

This reminder phrase is repeated over and over while tapping all the points. Do as many rounds of EFT as necessary until the movie is rated down to 1.

Tell the Movie Aloud

Whether you are working alone or with the help of a partner, verbally describe your movie. However, it would be necessary to interrupt the story each time you feel any emotional intensity to apply a treatment. Pausing the story to apply a treatment provides a golden opportunity to free yourself from unwanted negative emotions. This is contrary to standard counseling techniques, which call for the client to tell the whole story without any interruption. Tap on the different EFT points until you feel no intensity and then continue describing the following segment of your movie. Repeat the process each time you feel re-stimulated by its contents.

Re-Test Your Feelings About the Movie

Re-run the movie in your mind and apply the EFT treatment until you feel free of any negative emotion. This technique not only has the benefit of clearing us of any negative emotion attached to the situation we have worked on, but also its emotionally liberating effects are extended to other associated issues thus enhancing our life and helping us to grow.

The Narrative Technique

This is an extension of the Movie Technique. You could benefit from this technique when you are working on your emotional issues alone or with a partner. Select a specific emotionally charged event in your life and talk about it. Stop at the point of your story when you feel that your feelings of anxiety, anger, grief, or fear intensify. At that instance, apply the tapping sequence as necessary until they rate down to 1. Then resume your story.

After each pause, the subsequent narrative may take you to another aspect of the emotional issue you are clearing. The emerging aspects may have been forgotten, but the fact that they come back to your mind signifies that you have simply suppressed the emotions to protect yourself from the pain they may have caused. The following guidelines should be taken into consideration when applying this technique:

Rate the Intensity of the Story

Give your story a number from 1 to 10. If the intensity is high like 8 or 9 do some general tapping rounds to reduce the severity of it. Proceeding with general statements should help to reduce the intensity. For example:

"Even though I don't want to think about this story, ..."

"Even though I feel anxious just to think about this incident, ..."

Relate the Story from the General to the Specific

Once you feel that the intensity has decreased and you are more comfortable narrating the story, you can begin with a general introduction, something neutral, perhaps describing the place where the story took place, then proceed to describe the specific memory.

Stop to Apply a Treatment

For this technique to work it is essential that you stop to tap every time you feel any intensity. Usually it is difficult to break the narrative because we want to tell the story from the beginning to the end. Contrary to EFT, conventional psychological treatment encourages the patient to talk without interruption. If you do not stop at the emotionally charged points of the story, you will miss the opportunity to heal.

While tapping, repeat the segment of the story that triggered the emotional response as many times as necessary, until you feel totally at ease with it, not even a hint of hesitation or emotion.

Re-Test Your Feelings About the Story

With you eyes closed, visualize the situation with all of its details, paying attention to your feelings for any signs of distress. You are probably going to feel comfortable and free from any distress associated with the event, but if you do not, it means that you have discovered another aspect or underlying cause. Apply EFT to whatever comes up until you can talk about the whole event without feeling anything.

"The key to independence lies in knowing that at every moment, in every instance, we are creating our life. The more we acknowledge this truth, the more power and freedom we experience. Rather than blaming ourselves for the things we do not like in our life, we now realize we are manifesting our reality and have the power to change it."

Shakti Gawain

8.

APPLICATIONS OF EFT

Illustrative Cases

In this chapter I describe practical applications of EFT to clearing negative emotions, including phobias, anxiety, psychological trauma, and various addictions. They are drawn from my personal and professional experience in helping others. These cases illustrate the possible applications of EFT to improve our lives.

PHOBIAS

A phobia is an irrational, persistent, and uncontrollable fear that induces a compelling desire to avoid an object, activity, or situation that generates the fear. Most people who suffer from phobias consciously know their fear does not have a realistic foundation but nonetheless their fear is so real that in some instances it is incapacitating. Trembling, heart palpitations, headache, nausea, tears, sweaty palms, upset stomach and diarrhea are some of the symptoms phobia sufferers experience. The list of phobias can be endless, but some of the most common ones are the fear of public speaking (number one in America), insects, rodents, heights, needles, dogs, flying, water, darkness, closed or open spaces, speed, driving, etc.

EFT has shown to be an extraordinary technique to cure long term phobia sufferers. It does not matter the intensity of your phobia or the number of years you have had it. In some cases only one round of EFT is sufficient to be totally free from a phobia that has controlled your life for decades.

In my personal experience, I had the opportunity to test the results of EFT on my fear of needles. I use to be afraid of going for my yearly medical check up because I knew what was coming after that, the blood test. My hands became very cold, my breathing intensified, and I felt like fainting every time a blood sample was taken. The sight of the nurse getting ready to draw my blood paralyzed me with fear. It all started when I was a teenager and I had to go to the hospital suffering from food poisoning. An inexperienced nurse could not find the vain, and pinched my arm so many times that I ended up crying profusely. In the end, both of my arms had bruises and several haematomas. From that time my fear of needles began and through the years it only intensified. However, after I applied two EFT treatments, the fear disappeared completely. I applied the treatment when I was still in my car waiting to enter the lab. I pictured the nurse getting ready to draw my blood. The thought helped me connect with my fear and I rated its intensity to 7; then I used the following set up affirmation:

"Even though I feel the needle in my arm I am totally relaxed and calm."

After a round with this affirmation I felt better, the intensity was reduced to 3; I did another treatment of EFT saying:

"Even though I am still nervous about the entire procedure of having this blood test I choose to be relaxed"

It has been three years since I applied the treatment and the fear never returned, even though I have visited the lab several times since then. The original traumatic event has become just a memory and nothing else.

I have been able to help other people get rid of their phobias. One interesting case is that of a 68-year-old woman who was terrified of mice for decades. She heard me talking about the benefit of EFT but she was skeptical, but receptive. In her own words she said "I would give it a try. The only thing I have to loose is this panic." We started by attuning to the negative emotion. It was rated 10, very high. She had to do several rounds of EFT because there were many aspects of her fear that had to be eradicated. Some of the statements she used included a very general one at first:

"Even though I have this fear of mice, I completely accept myself."

She reported a decrease, but a negligible one; it went from 10 to 8. We explored the origin of her phobia and it went back to the time when her older sister, who always put her to sleep when she was little, frighten her saying that there was a dirty mouse who lived in their house and came out at night to bite the thumbs of little girls who were not sleeping. Her sister told her that she had to fall asleep fast to avoid the mouse. This woman believed that the mouse was a monster that was going to eat her. Her phobia had many components. She did several EFT rounds picturing in her mind the image she had about the mouse and alternatively used the following phrases:

"Even though the mouse is after me, I love and accept myself."

" Even though the mouse is going to eat me, I love and accept

myself."

"Even though my sister tricked me, I forgive her."

After that she reported feeling free of her fear. To test her feelings, she described in detailed the origin of her phobia and she did not report any negative emotions. We also used a picture of a mouse, which in the past made her feel very uncomfortable. This time she did not have any discomfort. For the final test, she decided to go to a pet shop to touch a mouse in a cage. She reported that now she was finally able to give her daughter the pet she always wanted, a little white mouse.

This is not an uncommon result. The Emotional Freedom Internet site (www.emofree.com) is filled with testimonies of people who have achieved total relief from their unfounded fears.

In another case, a 53-year-old woman reported a strong fear of kitchen food disposals. She could not trace this fear of any particular situation in her life but she said that she has always been afraid that her hand was going to be crushed by the blades. She recently built a new home and the kitchen had two sinks, one with a food disposal machine. She was so afraid of it that she did not want to get near it. She asked the builder to have the food disposal dismantled, but her husband disagreed because he thought it was very convenient and he used it all the time. He wanted to help her overcome this unjustified feeling and suggested to her that she should face her fear, but for her the mere thought of the blades and the sound of the disposal was enough to have her trembling. It only took two rounds for her to overcome her fear and to discover the origin of it. She worked with the following set up phrases:

"Even though I am afraid of losing my fingers in the food disposal, I love and accept myself."

"Even though I am so afraid of the food disposal, I love and accept myself."

After the two rounds of treatment, she reported having no fear at all. We tested it by asking her to imagine herself using the food disposal, and hearing the grinding noise the machine makes when it is in use. She felt no discomfort at all. She also said that while tapping a memory of herself when she was about eight came to her mind. She was helping her mother do the laundry in one of those old-fashioned washing machines equipped with rolling cylinders to press the wet clothing. While feeding the rollers with a garment, her arm was trapped and pressed. She momentarily panicked as she was certain that she was going to lose her arm. Hearing the screams, her mother rushed to stop the machine thus preventing a tragedy, but the intense fear remained in her unconscious mind.

It often happens that when we work on our negative emotions other images or events associated with them emerge into our conscious mind. Sometimes they include situations we did not know were there, like the one described above; they provide us with valuable information and an excellent opportunity to clear traumatic events in life.

ADDICTION

Addictions are characterized as an uncontrollable compulsion, a constant craving or the tendency to repeat a habit or behavior in spite of clear evidences of its harmful implications. In terms of EFT and TFT, addictions are considered the consequence of anxiety. Alcohol, drugs, food, tobacco, chocolate, coffee, tranquilizers, etc., are some of the substances sought by the addict as inducing a calming and relaxing effect, but the essence of the problem is that these substances or actions act as temporary relievers only. They conceal the real reason behind the addiction. When the effect of the substance passes anxiety appears again, thus perpetuating a continuous cycle that reenforces itself by the transitory calming effects it produces in the mind and body.

The use of EFT has proven to be very effective in eradicating addictions. By tackling the anxiety which is the underlying core behind all addictions, the driving force of the addition is permanently eliminated. I have extensive experience counseling clients with drug and alcohol dependency. I have seen the devastating effects these substances do to the life of my clients. Men, women, and adolescents who first started using these substances for curiosity, peer pressure, availability, or over exposure, become enslaved by an uncontrollable desire to consume them later in life.

Before knowing about EFT, I used regular counseling techniques. I explored the causes and consequences of their addiction, I used behavior modification, and a large array of other counseling techniques. I have seen many clients struggling to stop their addiction and genuinely trying to get rid of their negative behavior, relapsing again after sometime. Conventional therapies are only partially effective. Scientific literature uses a biological deterministic approach to explain the problem. Proponents of this theory argue that the cause of all addictions is biological and genetic in nature. Whether or not an addiction is inherited, EFT offers a new perspective as well as an innovative solution to eliminate the complex problem of addiction.

All types of addictions could be effectively treated with EFT. However, we need to emphasize that some addictions could require more intensive treatment than others. This is due to the fact that people struggling with a substance or behavioral addiction have strong defense mechanisms. They have to face the self-denial of the problem they have, and their internal resistance to change it.

This situation is compounded by the person's self-doubt about giving up an addiction when they have found that the substance or behavior addiction is the only constant companion and source of satisfaction in life. The addict would often have the following questions:

"What would I need to do to replace my addiction?"

"Would I have to develop new relationships with new friends and family and stop socializing with my current friends?"

"Am I strong enough to manage the withdrawal symptoms?"

David Rourke (www.davidrourke.ca) suggests that by answering all of these questions many issues will emerge and that tapping on those emerging issues is essential to overcoming the addiction. This could be a challenging endeavor. In order to achieve meaningful changes in our lives, we first need to recognize that we have a problem. We tend to use denial and resistance as defense mechanisms to avoid facing any changes. If you find yourself facing this situation, working with an experienced EFT specialist is advisable. If people in your circle regularly tell you that they are concerned with your behavior and habits, but you do not seem to agree with them or you simply do not perceive yourself as having any problem that you cannot control, this is an indication of denial.

A useful strategy outline by David Rourke consists in making a list of all the positive and negative aspects of keeping your addiction, as well as the positive and negative aspects of giving up the addiction. This exercise will bring issues for EFT treatments.

EFT successfully reduces the distress associated with withdrawal symptoms. These symptoms have physical and emotional consequences. EFT eliminates the craving and drastically decreases the anxiety, because cravings are caused by a desire to reduce an anxiety. To eliminate your addiction, whatever it may be, apply EFT treatments to the cravings. For instance, if alcohol is the substance you are addicted to you could apply a treatment while using the following phrases:

"Even though I am craving for a drink right now, I love and accept myself."

"Even though I feel this urge to have a beer, I love and accept myself."

"Even though alcohol has always been my companion, I love and accept myself."

"Even though alcohol makes me forget about my pain, I now choose to accept myself."

"Even though I feel that alcohol controls my life, I now chose to stop drinking."

"Even though my drinking has caused so much pain to me as well as other people, I chose to forgive myself and to stop drinking."

"Even though I feel that alcohol controls my life, I love and accept

myself."

"Even though I feel that once I have started drinking I cannot stop, I love and accept myself."

"Even though I want to use alcohol when things are (not) going well in my life, I love and accept myself."

All of these affirmations acknowledge the addiction at the same time that they create self acceptance. Some affirmations offer a statement of choice. You can use any of these affirmations by substituting the alcohol for the substance or behavior you are addicted to. EFT is an exceptional technique that can be used any time addictive cravings come to the surface. As with any other EFT treatments, watch for ideas or feelings, or memories that emerge while tapping and apply treatments to the new feelings or memories after you finish the current one.

Many people have reported rapid success in eliminating coffee, chocolate, soft drinks, and sweets addiction with only a few rounds of tapping. However, addiction to drugs and alcohol may take a longer and more persistent approach. Craig recommends to apply the basic steps of EFT twenty-five times per day to keep the level of anxiety and the cravings under control, as well as to overpower the effects of Psychological Reversal. We discussed psychological reversal in the previous chapter and described it as the major block behind many addictions.

It is recommended to create a routine that will help you remember to apply EFT treatments throughout the day. For instance, write reminder note to yourself and place them around the house and in your car. When you find a card, apply a treatment at once; it only takes a few minutes. Some of my alcohol-dependent clients report that the most difficult time they confront are those occasions in which everyone is drinking, the ambiance is favorable, and the smell of their favorite substance stimulates them. I always suggest to my clients to avoid those situations in which alcohol is present, and to stay away from people who encourage or condone their addiction. Although, these recommendations are sound and helpful, sometimes it is difficult to avoid dangerous environments. In those situations, when the craving is strong, an EFT treatment should take care of the urges. This is equally applicable to any other addictive substance or behavior: any time you feel an urge to satisfy an addictive behavior, apply an EFT treatment.

Now that you have learned to overcome the withdrawal symptoms and the cravings, you have the tools to control your addictive behavior. However, to completely conquer the addiction itself, you would need to become aware of those specific events or situations that led you to develop and maintain your addictive behavior. For instance, smokers tend to light up a cigarette when a specific situation makes them nervous or anxious (e.g., a meeting, an interview, an argument, a decision to be made, having to wait for someone or something, etc.). Some people may say that they only smoke to relax, after a meal, or a cup of coffee, or at a social event, but if someone needs a cigarette to relax is because something is making them nervous or uneasy, otherwise what would be the reason? Applying an EFT treatment to the core of those specific events that create the anxiety is important, but it could be challenging because you may or may not be aware of those events.

If that is the case, Gary Craig recommends an excellent emotional cleansing exercise. It involves making an exhaustive list of all the specific events that have been troublesome in your life and clearing the negative emotion associated with each of them through EFT treatments until you feel the events have no impact on your life any longer. Be alert that while you are doing this emotional work, other events that you thought you had forgotten may come to your conscious mind. This implies that you have to clear the emotions associated with the event. I recommend to set aside a time for this emotional cleansing and to have a notebook to take notes of all the particular events that will emerge. This not only will help you overcome the addictive behavior, but also will help you physically and emotionally by finding peace within yourself and with your surroundings.

The following case reflects the use of EFT on a cigarette smoker who had been addicted for over twenty-three years. Laura smoked a pack of cigarettes a day as a way to relax as well as to control her emotions. At work she took regular "smoking breaks" during the day. The health institution where she works wanted to promote a better environment and was giving special incentives to those employees who quit their smoking addiction. Laura felt pressured to stop smoking at work and at home. Her husband did not allow her to smoke in the house or in the car when their new baby was present. Laura had tried several times to quit with different methods, but nothing seemed to work. She was very concerned about suffering the withdrawal symptoms. She heard about EFT and wanted to try it. The first step was to determine the compelling emotions behind her cigarette dependency. We did some exploratory work and I asked her to give me a list of all the positive and negative aspects of quitting cigarette smoking. Amongst the positive aspects she mentioned:

- Improve her health and avoid developing cancer.

- Saving money.

- Avoiding family conflict.

■   Avoiding unpleasant smell in her hair, clothing, and home.

■   Improving her sense of taste.

Amongst the negative aspects of quitting, she came up with an extensive list, including the following:

■   Suffering the withdrawal symptoms.

■   Missing the social aspect of smoking with friends and colleagues.

■   Not being able to relax without it.

■   Gaining body weight.

We applied several EFT treatments by tapping on her identified fears. Each treatment was done while repeating the following affirmations:

"Even though I am afraid of the withdrawal symptoms, I love and accept myself."

"Even though I am afraid to make the commitment to stop smoking, I accept and forgive myself."

"Even though I feel that I wouldn't know what to do without my cigarettes, I love and accept myself."

"Even though I felt very much part of the group when I was 15 and Ruth taught me how to smoke, I now choose to take the steps to socialize without smoking a cigarette."

"Even though when I was 15, I smoked to be accepted by the group,

I now choose to believe that I don't need to smoke to be accepted by others because I accept and love myself free from the smoking habit."

"Even though I am afraid that if I stop smoking at work I will have problems thinking straight, I now choose to trust my intellectual capacity and my strength."

After the treatments Laura reported that the thought of going through the day without a cigarette did not make her anxious as it used to. She remarked that she felt relaxed and confident about the thought of quitting. However, she had some apprehensions about facing the withdrawal symptoms. We then tapped on the following affirmations:

"Even though I feel very anxious without smoking, I deeply and completely accept myself."

"Even though I feel very hungry without my cigarettes to help me go through the day, I deeply and completely accept myself."

"Even though I want to be part of the smoking group at work, I deeply and completely accept myself."

"Even though I am afraid of gaining weight as I did the last time I tried to stop smoking, I love and accept myself."

"Even though I feel angry at my husband for wanting to control my smoking addiction, I accept myself."

We worked through all of her emotions associated with giving up smoking as well as on all of the withdrawal symptoms. We extensively tapped on specific situations that were associated with the time when she started smoking twenty-three years ago.

Issues of acceptance, self-appreciation, and assertiveness.

I advised Laura to tap on her own to get through the cravings, to pay attention to her emotions, and to tap on them. One month later she confided that she did not have the desire to smoke anymore. She said that she wanted to share a secret with me. She told me that even though she has worked intensely on her emotions and cravings all of this time, for about two weeks she kept a pack of cigarettes hidden in a drawer, just in case, but she decided that she did not want to smoke anymore, and threw it in the garbage. She keeps tapping on her own for whatever emotional situation comes up. She found the technique very powerful and reported that for the first time in her life she has gone for about four months without smoking. She has not relapsed and she feels very strongly that this time the quitting is for life. The key to Laura's success was the work she did to discover the emotional reasons behind her addiction. Once this was done, EFT effectively removed the unwanted energy associated with them.

TRAUMA

Trauma is a normal reaction to an unnatural event that can be interpreted as a condition of the body or mind caused by severe injury or shock. It is the constant or sporadic effect of unprocessed internal messages and impressions formed during a critical life event. These messages can develop from any experience that leaves us feeling threatened. However, it is not the event or situation that determines whether something is traumatic to us or not, but instead it is our own perception of the event. This explains the reason why when two people are exposed exactly to the same traumatic event, such as a serious automobile accident, they may react in different ways. One may carry the trauma for years not being able to drive a car for the rest of his life, while the others remember the accident but have no negative emotions associated with it.

According to EFT postulates, a trauma or negative emotion causes an interference in the body's energy system. To eliminate the emotional impact of a trauma, we need to free that negative energy associated with it.

Unresolved traumas can have physical, emotional, and intellectual consequences. Some of the symptoms of emotional trauma include chronic physical pain, feelings of helplessness, sleep dysfunction, nightmares, depression, anxiety, obsessive behaviors, nervousness, hopelessness, anger and resentment, emotional numbness, sexual dysfunctions, memory lapses, mood swings, or vivid recurring memories of the traumatic experience. All of these symptoms and many more physical and emotional problems that are associated with traumatic memories can be resolved through EFT. Persistence is essential to the total elimination of traumatic reactions. EFT does not eliminate the memory of the traumatic event, only the negative energy attached to it. Once that negative energy is released, the recollections of the traumatic events would no longer have the emotional strength they had. What follows is a depiction of the effective use of EFT on a childhood traumatic experience.

Tamika was a very quiet eighteen-year-old. Her parents brought her to counseling because they were concerned about her shyness, silent, and friendless behavior. She was unable to initiate social interaction with other people. She was distracted, indifferent toward her school work, and uninterested in anything except her books and her music.

While talking to Tamika, I noticed that she only had problems socializing with children her own age. She stated that she wanted to be more sociable but she did not know how. She was also afraid of being rejected and she cited that as the reason for keeping to herself and not initiating any conversation with her peers. Tamika started Montessori school at the age of three and did not have these problems then. Her difficulties relating to her peers developed later on while she studied at that same school. In the beginning she had a group of boys she always played with and felt very loved and accepted by them. She remained at the same school, with the same group of children, for about nine years. She took six months off to travel with her parents and when she returned the entire social dynamic was different. Some of the boys in her pervious group rejected her and so did most of the girls due to the fact that they did not see Tamika as one of them because she preferred to play with boys.

Through EFT we discovered the core issue that had affected Tamika for many years. A very traumatic experience that had deeply influenced her life: during the first half of the school day, the children had a discussion circle called Agenda Time. The classroom had a box placed in one corner of the room where the children were encouraged to write the name of a person they were having problems with for open discussion with the group.

In the meeting, all thirty children sat in a circle, the box was placed in the middle of the group, and someone picked the paper with the name of the student in question. The complaint was presented to the entire class and the child who was in the agenda had the opportunity to stand up and explain his/her actions. With the teacher's input, the group would arrive at a solution.

Tamika's name was called. She was being accused of stealing color markers from other students. Tamika knew that she has not done such a thing, but several of the girls who disliked her conspired to say that they had seen her stealing and that they had markers missing. Tamika felt very confused, the teacher asked every student in the circle if they have had color markers missing, and some of them said yes to agree with the popular girls. During Tamika's recollection of the event, she remembers that three boys said that they have never seen Tamika taking anything from others. But while Tamika was being judged, she remembered an occasion during the school year when she took one pencil from the lost-and-found box. Then the teacher asked her if she had taken pencils from other students. Feeling very confused and yielding into peer pressure, she said yes. As a punishment, Tamika was asked to take out of her drawer all of her own new color markers, put them in a box and pass them around the circle. Every child was asked to search through Tamika's box and they were instructed by the teacher to take any marker they wanted from Tamika's box as a way of paying back for the ones she allegedly took from them. While they were picking through her box, she was asked to stand up and give an apology to the class.

Tamika knew that she had never taken any thing from the other children, except for the pencil she took from the lost-and-found box when she could not find her own, but the fact that several of her classmates were incriminating her confused her and made her admit to wrong doing. Feeling humiliated and ashamed from the experiance, she cried inconsolably knowing that she was the object of a tremendous injustice. She remembers not being able to stop crying for the rest of the day. At the end of the day, several of the girls that had accused her wrote her a letter apologizing for what they did to her. They said that they were sorry they made that story up and they asked for forgiveness.

Tamika remembered the incident with vivid detail. While she was describing it, we stopped several times to tap. We worked on issues of trust, embarrassment, self-respect, honesty, power, friendship, victimization, and guilt. Every time she described the event her feelings were less and less intense. During the counseling session, EFT treatments were specifically applied to the memory of each of the children that had abused her, and the things they said and did to her. These were some of the EFT affirmations used in the process:

"Even though I felt so vulnerable during Agenda Time standing up in front of the group and admitting to something that I didn't do, I love and forgive myself."

"Even though Ms. Smith and all of the children thought that I had done something wrong, I forgive myself for not speaking up and defending myself."

"Even though I felt so humiliated when Laura, Mary, Samantha and the rest of the class took advantage of the situation to grab my best markers, I forgive myself for allowing that to happen."

"Even though I feel so much pain for the way I was treated when I was only a little girl, I love and accept myself."

"Even though Laura and Marlene apologized for what they did to me I am still angry at them for blaming me for something I didn't do."

"Even though I am very angry at Ms. Smith for the way she handled the situation, I love and accept myself."

"Even though I learned to mistrust everybody, I now choose to give people a chance to get to know me."

"Even though Laura and the other girls apologized to me for what they did, I forgive myself for not bringing that note to Agenda Time

to clear up my name and to get my markers back."

"I love and accept myself and I forgive Ms. Smith and all of the students for what they did to me."

"I love and forgive myself for accepting responsibility and blaming myself for something I didn't do."

"I now choose to speak up and let people know how I am and what I think."

"I love and accept myself and I am now open to the possibility of letting other people get to know me."

"I love and accept myself and I am now choosing to take the initiative to trust other people."

At the end of the two-hour session, Tamika was able to talk about the incident without any emotion attached to it. She now sees it as un unfortunate event that had held her down for many years, keeping her from trusting others and herself. The last time she contacted me she mentioned that there are other issues she needs to work on but the good news was that she is making wonderful progress in letting others know who she is. She is also expressing her opinion and points of view in class as well as in informal conversation; she is making new friends and trusting them more. Last time she saw me she said "with my 'new self' everything seems to be easier; I have even found a nice boyfriend with whom I feel very comfortable."

Tamika's memory about the incident is still with her. EFT does not eradicate the memory of the event but it eliminates the negative emotions attached to it. Now she can talk about the school incident without tears as if it never had any influence on her life. She sees the incident as something unfortunate that happened in her life but nothing else.

ANXIETY

Everyone has experienced a certain degree of anxiety from time to time. This can be considered a normal fact of life. For instance, we feel anxious when we are at work and have to meet a deadline, take a test, go for a job interview, or give a presentation. Certain amount of anxiety is considered useful by the National Institute of Mental Health and the American Psychological Association because it can make us more alert or careful. A bit of anxiety helps us concentrate and do a better job. It can also protect us when we are in a crowded city and we are advised to be attentive to our belongings, or when we walk along in a dark street. A normal state of temporary anxiety usually ends after we are out of the stressful situation. However, the National Institute of Health has reported that millions of Americans live in a constant state of anxiety. This has been shown as a constant and persistent emotional problem that does not go away and gets even worse over time. Some of the symptoms include:

- Fatigue.

- Difficulty sleeping.

- Irritability.

- Feeling on the edge.

- Difficulty concentrating.

- Symptoms associated with muscle tension, such as

trembling, feeling shaky, muscle aches and soreness.

■ Physical symptoms, such as sweaty hands, dry mouth, nausea, diarrhea, need to urinate frequently, trouble swallowing, etc.

Persistent and untreated anxiety can degenerate into a variety of diseases and debilitating conditions. Until now, the standard treatment recommended for this condition consisted of medications, therapy, or a combination of both. Medicine only temporarily relieves the symptoms . With EFT it is possible to eliminate the cause of anxiety. Thus, EFT indeed offers the possibility of a permanent cure. It is a treatment that you can apply to your self not only to control the everyday stresses of life, but also to treat all the conditions mentioned above. However, for complex emotional problems with extensive emotional ramifications the assistance of an experienced EFT practitioner would be extremely valuable.

Anna approached me because of her problem with ongoing anxiety. She was complaining of feeling a constant state of tension with physical symptoms that included a sharp pain in her right arm, heart palpitation, and shaky legs. Her symptoms intensified when she was in crowded places. She complained that her condition has forced her to change her life. She used to have an extroverted personality, very friendly and outgoing. Every Friday she used to go out dancing; she used to have an intense social life. On the contrary, Anna now hides behind her work and she gets increasingly anxious towards the end of the week when her friends call to invite her out. She no longer answers the telephone and doesn't even want to go grocery shopping for the fear of facing all of the symptoms.

We started by exploring the origin of her anxiety and

seeking any particular incident associate with it. She said that it all began about six months ago when she was going out to meet a friend for dinner, two men approached her pretending to need help in finding an address stole her purse, and threatened her with a gun if she didn't cooperate. It all happened in the middle of a crowded street, but nobody helped. After the incident, she had constant fear and anxiety that she would be robed again and she fears every man that crosses her way. Her friends often advise her to face her fears and to overcome the incident. They tell her that the possibility of something like that occurring again is slim, that the city is relatively safe, and that she should regain her trust, but she feels that no one understands her.

We started treatment by using the Narrative Technique. She went over the incident and stopped to tap every time she felt any intensity. She recounted the story until she felt no emotion attached to it. We worked on the incident using the following setup statements:

"I love and accept myself, even though I am facing all of these symptoms."

"I love and accept myself, even though I am very afraid I may be robbed again."

"I love and accept myself, even though I feel guilty for trusting those people."

"Even though these men had a gun and wanted to hurt me, I choose to live my life without fear."

"Even though I was victimized by those men and felt very helpless, I now choose to take my power back."

"Even though I felt helpless and weak, I now choose to feel safe and secure, relaxed and calm as I regain my trust in others."

"Even though I feel afraid to go out with my friends, I now choose to get my social life back as I feel protected at all times."

"I love and accept myself and I now choose to live without fear."

Before the treatment, the level of distress was rated as 8. The intensity level started dropping after a few sessions and came down to 2. She said she still had some of the physical symptoms. We tapped addressing the physical symptoms directly.

"Even though my heart feels that it wants to get out of my chest, I now choose to feel relaxed, secure, and totally safe."

"Even though my legs are shaky, I trust them to take me anywhere I want, as I feel safe and secure wherever I go."

Anna also worked diligently on her own with a list of affirmations we developed together and she reported excellent recovery. Two months after our last session, she indicated that she has started going out with her friends again; she is not afraid of the telephone anymore, and does not avoid answering it. She feels safe and secure, she takes her normal precautions in the street, but does not feel threatened. All of her physical symptoms have disappeared. In her own words she said "I feel like myself again."

"When your life simply becomes a joy from moment to moment, a dance from moment to moment, when your life is nothing but a festival of lights, then each moment is precious because once it is gone, it is gone forever."

Osho.

"Just trust yourself, then you will know how to live."

Goethe.

REFERENCES

American Psychological Association.<www.apa.org>

Callahan, Roger. 2001. Tapping the Healer Within. Contemporary Books Chicago, IL.

Craig, Gary. Emotional Freedom Techniques. <www.emofree.com>

Eden, D., and Feinstein, D., 1998. Energy Medicine. Tarcher/Putnam, New York, NY.

Forem, J. and Shimer, S., 1999. Healing with Pressure Points Therapy. Prentice Hall Press, New York, NY.

Lecrubier, Y., Clerc, G., Didi, R., and Kieser, M., 2002. Efficacy of St. John's Wort Extract WS 5570 in Major Depression: A Double-Blind, Placebo-Controlled Trial. Am J. Psychiatry 159:1361-1366.

National Institute of Mental Health. <www.nimh.nih.gov>

Rourke, David. 2007, <www.davidrourke.ca>

Sahelian, R., 2007. St. John's Wort Information. A Discussion of St. John's Wort for depression and St. John's Wort Side Effects. www.raysahelian.com/stjohn.html

Serrano, S.E., 2007. The Three Spirits. SpiralPress, Ambler, PA.

Swingle, P.G.., Pulos, L., and Swingle, M.K. 2004. Neurophysiological indicators of EFT treatment of post-traumatic stress. Subtle Energies and Energy

Medicine, 15, l, 75-86.

Teeguarden, I.M., 1978. Acupressure Way of Health: jin shin do. Japan Publications, Inc., Tokyo, Japan.

Wells, S., Polglase, K., Andrews, H., Carrington, P., & Baker, A.H. (2003). Evaluation of a Meridian-Based Intervention, Emotional Freedom Techniques (EFT), for Reducing Specific Phobias of Small Animals. Journal of Clinical Psychology, 59 (9). 943-966

Wood, Stephanie. <www.emofree.com> April 2007 News Letter.

INDEX

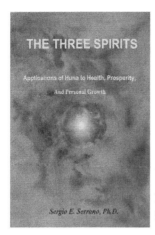

THE THREE SPIRITS

Applications of Huna to Health, Prosperity, and Personal Growth

Sergio E. Serrano, Ph.D.

"If you are not using Huna, you are working too hard."

Max Freedom Long, author of The Secret Science Behind Miracles

Huna means "secret" in the Hawaiian language. It refers to the coded knowledge of the ancient Kahunas, who were known for healing the sick, controlling the weather, walking over hot lava, and predicting and changing the future. You can use the principles of Huna to improve your health, better your finances, increase wealth, acquire material possessions you desire, achieve personal and professional objectives, enrich your relationship with others, and enhance the overall quality of life. Perhaps you have used visualization before, but do not know why sometimes it does not work. Know the forces and meet the entities of your mind that control the art of mental creation. Develop and use the skills necessary to effectively and efficiently achieve your desires.

Huna techniques are combined with Thought Field Therapy (TFT) and Emotional Freedom Techniques (EFT). TFT/EFT methods are based on energy therapies similar to acupuncture. They have been shown to effectively remove deep psychological fixations, complexes, fears, anxiety, phobias, and negative emotions, without the need of expensive "talk therapies."

Written in a simple style, the book includes many practical exercises and illustrations designed to gradually develop and apply the principles.

About the Author: Dr. Sergio E. Serrano is an engineer, scientist, and university professor. He is an example of the wave of scientists increasingly interested in studying psychic phenomena from a rigorous point of view.

Published by:
SpiralPress
1217 Charter Lane
Ambler, PA 19002
E-mail: hydroscience@earthlink.net
http://home.earthlink.net/~hydroscience

AN ART OF LIVING

André Maurois

Our lives are works of art, expressions of inner beauty, conceived and created by our inner selves, tested by the circumstances and experiences of life, perfected and modified by the learning and growth resulting from these experiences. Few authors have expressed these timeless principles with more eloquence than André Maurois (1885 - 1967), one of the most celebrated and prolific French writers of the 20th century.

An Art of Living was first published in France in 1939. It is divided into five sections: The Art of Thinking, The Art of Loving, The Art of Working, The Art of Leadership, and The Art of Growing Old. Each section contains very profound, timeless, wisdom about the most important aspects we face in life. The real value of An Art of Living, is that the sentences are not merely a collection of words to convey a practical thought, but a communication to the spirit of the reader. Maurois speaks to the soul of the reader. The principles he conveys remain as valid and as useful in the 21st century as they were in the 20th.

There is so much insight in this book! Maurois accurately predicts the ultimate failure of all social revolutions; the necessity of slow change in human customs and attitudes as a key to lasting changes; the technological development and implementation of robots in large assembly lines; the characteristics of a reasonable and effective government; the inner virtues to cultivate in order to successfully overcome the adversities of life; the qualities to seek in order to maintain stable, loving, relationships; the attributes to encourage as an effective manager; the essentials by which to plan a long and enjoyable retirement; and the principles behind an effective educational system. The book speaks to young and old alike. An Art of Living remained out of print for several decades. This new translation by Sergio E. Serrano intends to resurrect this little treasure of a book for the English readers of today; it remains faithful to the original French edition and to the style of the author.

Published by:
SpiralPress
1217 Charter Lane
Ambler, PA 19002
E-mail: hydroscience@earthlink.net
http://home.earthlink.net/~hydroscience

1279064

Made in the USA